BIGGER PETE

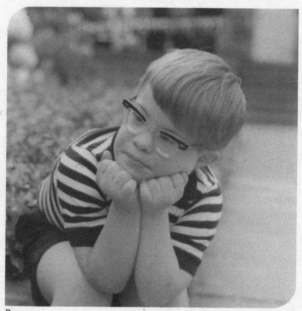

Pete

Bigger Pete

Conversations Between
Life and Afterlife

Elizabeth Bodien

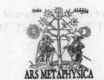

ARS METAPHYSICA

an imprint of Sunbury Press, Inc.
Mechanicsburg, PA USA

ARS METAPHYSICA

an imprint of Sunbury Press, Inc.
Mechanicsburg, PA USA

For information about special discounts for bulk purchases, please contact Sunbury Press Orders Dept. at (855) 338-8359 or orders@sunburypress.com.

To request one of our authors for speaking engagements or book signings, please contact Sunbury Press Publicity Dept. at publicity@sunburypress.com.

FIRST ARS METAPHYSICA EDITION: June 2023

Set in Adobe Garamond | Interior design by Crystal Devine | Cover by Darleen Sedjro | Edited by Sarah Peachey.

Publisher's Cataloging-in-Publication Data
Names: Bodien, Elizabeth, author.
Title: Bigger Pete : conversations between life and afterlife / Elizabeth Bodien.
Description: First trade paperback edition. | Mechanicsburg, PA : Ars Metaphysica, 2023.
Summary: Alzheimer's Disease causes Pete to lose the ability to speak and understand others. So how is his sister talking to him? When Pete was asleep, Elizabeth Bodien was in hypnotic trance, doing automatic writing. *Bigger Pete* is a memoir about communicating with a sibling over the last eight years of his life—and into the afterlife.
Identifiers: ISBN : 978-1-62006-897-7 (papberback) | ISBN : 979-8-88819-105-7 (ePub).
Subjects: BODY, MIND & SPIRIT / Afterlife & Reincarnation | HEALTH & FITNESS / Diseases / Alzheimer's & Dementia | FAMILY & RELATIONSHIPS / Siblings.

Product of the United States of America
0 1 1 2 3 5 8 13 21 34 55

Continue the Enlightenment!

Dedicated to Pete, Bigger Pete,
and all our bigger selves

BROTHER AND SISTER

Two children stand at edge of a wailing sea,
yearning full for it, and for what else,
they do not know. Together he and she
lean into wind, remembering father, mother.
They're holding hands, eyes closed, and feeling free.
The storm turns wild; it scares both sister, brother.
Ferocious night, the world seems near its end
right here, right now, where these two children stand.

Black waves stretch, frothing white to distant stars.
The last grass on this cliff lies trampled down.
The wind swirls chords as if from crazed guitars
that stir up moans from stones that sprawl around.
The world is wasted, naught but scum and scars,
and in this maelstrom, two, at least, will drown.
The children search each other's eyes in fear,
not knowing what approaches soon or near.

To a guild without a name, these two belong,
in time but who don't follow time's fast rule.
Each clenches hands in pockets to feel strong
against the forces, once kind, now turned cruel.
They wonder what they ever did so wrong.
(None of this was taught at home or school.)
Dark eye of storm eclipses in their eyes.
The finish of their fate conceals its whys.

—Elizabeth Bodien, 2013

CONTENTS

CONTENTS

VOICES IN THE CONVERSATIONS

THOSE LIVING ON EARTH

Pete/Bro: A man with Down Syndrome and Alzheimer's disease

Elizabeth/Sis: Pete's sister

THOSE IN SPIRIT

Pete/Bro/Bigger Pete

Mom: Deceased mother of Pete and Elizabeth

Dad: Deceased father of Pete and Elizabeth

Putty: Nickname for a deceased American poet, gatekeeper to the world of spirit

Aunt Elizabeth: Mom's sister and Elizabeth's namesake

Unidentified spirits/Unidentified voices: Unnamed voices, often appearing here as a group

PART I

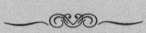

LIFE

CHAPTER ONE

THE TROUBLES BEGIN AND PUPPETS APPEAR

This is the story of Pete and me, at least some of the story. Who could ever tell all?

I am Elizabeth. Pete is my brother. Is he still my brother?

PETE'S BIRTH

In the 1950s, when our mother was expecting, we didn't know, before the birth, whether the baby would be a boy or a girl. And we certainly had no idea that this baby, our baby, would be someone special. Dad came from the hospital to tell us four older siblings that we had a new brother. We were excited and eager to see him. When the new baby came home from the hospital, we were not allowed to see him. Instead, there was a hush, and closed doors, and secrets. What was going on? Why couldn't we meet our new little brother?

We soon found out. Mom and Dad called us together. They explained that our new baby brother had something called Down syndrome, a genetic disorder caused by a third copy of the twenty-first chromosome. Down syndrome often results in slow physical growth, degrees of intellectual disability, and certain facial characteristics, as well as other less obvious traits. Mom and Dad told us our new brother looked a little different and that he would have problems. We didn't know what to think or feel about this. When we saw him, he did look a bit different, but we couldn't see any problems. The doctors had advised Mom and Dad to put the baby away in an institution and forget about him. But Mom and Dad were having none of that. He was family and would stay with family. His name would be Peter.

Once the initial shock about Down syndrome wore off, Mom went into high gear, taking it upon herself to learn all she could and to do everything she could to help Pete. Our new brother would need extra help. And we were the ones to give him that help.

PETE'S CHILDHOOD

Pete was a good-natured kid. He liked music and stories. When he was little, he could sit for hours looking through storybooks. When we would read to him, he memorized the words in his favorite stories. Every time, you would have to read the words exactly because he would correct you if you slipped up. And he would always say yes to a lullaby at bedtime.

As Pete grew, we could see that he did need extra help with dressing, eating, a lot of things. At our family dinner table, I always sat on Pete's right, his right arm near my left arm. Pete was not a neat eater and often ate with his hands. But he was affectionate, the more-hugs-the-better kind of affectionate. All that touching meant that by the time we finished dinner, the left sleeve of my clothes would always have some of Pete's dinner deposited there by his affectionate touches. I didn't like his messing up my clothes, but I tried not to let it bother me.

Being out in public with Pete was more difficult. One time we went swimming at a public swimming pool. The other children pointed at Pete, making unkind remarks. I felt angry at those children and defensive of Pete. At the same time, I could understand why they might question his looks or behavior. He was different. I was confused about what I should say or do. And I didn't notice, at the time, the effects of their taunts on Pete. It seemed to me that I should have understood him better, that we could have had a closer relationship, but I didn't know yet how to do that.

One thing Mom impressed on the rest of us was a sense of duty toward Pete, that we should help him whenever we could and teach him whenever we could. I took her advice seriously and did my best to help and teach Pete. As a result, when I would babysit kids in the neighborhood, their parents would call me again to babysit, saying they liked that I didn't just sit and watch TV but invented teaching games for the children, as I had been taught.

Pete was naturally sociable. He also seemed to have a strong inner life of his own. He took his own time to work out things for himself.

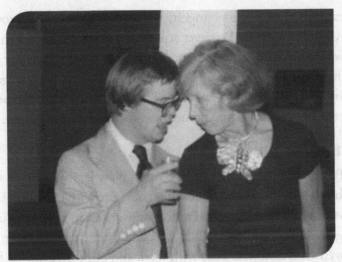

Pete and Mom, 1977.

It seemed much of what he learned and noticed around him he kept to himself, probably to some extent because it was difficult for him to express himself easily. It took longer for Pete to learn new things, and his speech was not clear. People who didn't know him sometimes couldn't understand him. We, too, had trouble understanding him at times. It could be quite frustrating.

One time he was trying to make himself understood and it just wasn't happening. At last, he stopped speaking. Then, exasperated, very slowly and carefully, one letter at a time, he spelled out his word: H–O–R–S–E. We were surprised because we hadn't realized he had already learned how to spell. Now we all had a tool when conversation alone didn't work. The spelling didn't always work that well, either, but it did help.

PETE GOES AWAY TO SCHOOL

We lived in an old red brick house in Rochester, New York. At that time, there was no school nearby that could accommodate those with disabilities. So, Pete left home, at just ten years old, to go to school far away in New Jersey, a special school for people with disabilities.

We visited him at his school. Those visits were not easy for me. Seeing Pete was wonderful, but I was confused about what to say or do with the other students at the school who had a variety of disabilities. On vacations, Pete came back home to Rochester.

Because Pete was the youngest, we older siblings were growing up and leaving home while Pete was still very young. When I went to college, I wanted to study the Japanese language, so that meant my going to the University of California at Berkeley, one of only four colleges at the time with such a language department. Being far away on the other side of the country, I didn't come home much or see Pete very often.

PETE BEGINS WORK

When Pete finished school, he stayed on in New Jersey, living in specially staffed houses and working at jobs open to those with disabilities. He did office work and especially liked when he worked in a greenhouse. Our family gathered on holidays when we could, even though the rest of us had moved away and were busy with work and our own growing families.

Suddenly and unexpectedly, Dad died of a heart attack. Pete was nineteen. Mom, who had been the mainstay in Pete's life all these years, continued to keep a close presence and involvement with him well into her elder years. Mom arranged for us three remaining siblings to serve as legal guardians for Pete when she passed on. Sadly, one sister had died in a car crash, leaving behind an infant daughter.

Eventually, I moved back east and started teaching. I lived within easy driving range of Pete and became more involved with his life. We spent holidays together and I became better acquainted with the people and community where he lived.

MOM FALLS ILL

Mom got Alzheimer's disease. I saw her decline, become less able to function. She needed more and more care. I would sit with her, those hours increasingly silent. When she spoke, she would tell me that when she tried to think of things, she sensed her mind going empty. She took medication for Alzheimer's, but little by little, she disappeared from herself. Sometimes she would ask for me even though I was sitting right there with her. She didn't recognize me. After declining with the disease for several years, she passed away at age eighty-seven.

We older siblings became Pete's legal guardians. He was fifty years old. Pete had been rather independent and liked living alone. He did his own laundry and cleaning and kept up his personal hygiene. But then he stopped shaving, cooking, and cleaning. He was confused occasionally and was beginning to forget things. He had more trouble expressing himself. He might start to say something, then mumble, "Try again," and re-start his sentence. These changes were ascribed to depression, a response to our mother's recent passing. I lived geographically closer to Pete than my sister and other brother did, so I spent more time with Pete, visiting him, going to meetings concerning his care, attending doctors' appointments with him, and bringing him to visit with us.

Pete, who before had insisted on his living by himself, agreed to have a roommate. Then, when he was fifty-three, he moved from the house he shared with his roommate to the supervised residences where he continued to live for many years.

PETE'S DIAGNOSIS

I was away for a few days at a conference in Florida when Pete's doctor called with the news that he was prescribing a medication because Pete was showing early signs of Alzheimer's disease. Having seen our mother struggle and succumb to Alzheimer's, I was devastated when I heard the news that Pete, only fifty-four years old, possibly had it too. What would Alzheimer's disease be like for Pete? Would Pete go through what my mother went through? People with Down syndrome have a high risk for Alzheimer's disease and often get it at an earlier age than other people. I didn't know then how Pete's experience would turn out to be different from our mother's experience.

I had been on the faculty at a community college where I taught cultural anthropology. However, I had retired early so that I could be more available to help as needed with Pete. The director of the group home where Pete was living said he could continue to live there unless his nursing needs exceeded what they were licensed and able to provide. I began to look for facilities closer to me where he could move to when the time came for that.

I was accepted into a low-residency MFA program to study poetry which required my being on campus in Colorado and far from Pete but for only two weeks each summer. So, my time and attention were divided between the poetry program and Pete. It was now three years past his diagnosis of Alzheimer's disease. He began showing more obvious signs of the disease—withdrawal from social activities, unusual irritability, more trouble with speaking, and, sadly, the loss of his delightful, dry sense of humor. For a snapshot of Pete at this time, I will add in here the report I wrote up of one of Pete's regular visits when he came to stay with us in Pennsylvania:

— Pete's Visit March 2013 —

We went to pick Pete up on Friday. He was full of hugs and all packed and ready. He had his suitcase (somehow missing socks, toilet articles, and a shaver), his packets of meds, and a big box of topical ointments. I asked the staff if there was anything new that I should know of. No.

On the drive to Pennsylvania, he stayed awake the whole way instead of nodding off, as he did more often now. We had packed both his walker and wheelchair. Happily, we didn't need the wheelchair at all. Even the walker got little use inside the house as he walked without it by holding on to walls when he needed to. His mobility was much better than on his November visit (when he seemed to be having a severe reaction to the drug Risperdal).

He still chooses to move as little as possible, though, and eschews any suggestions to go for a walk. He has his favorite chair in the kitchen, which he heads to as soon as he comes into the house. In the sunroom, he sits on the big wooden bench by the window to look at the newspaper, at least his favorite sports and weather pages. At dinner, he sits in the same place at the table. We maintain all of this routine more consciously now as the familiarity seems to be helpful. Also, I posted in his bedroom and on the kitchen fridge the schedule of meals that he keeps normally. We try to keep that when he visits, again for the comfort of familiar routine.

The sticking point always seems to be his showers. He has such an aversion to taking a shower. Friday night, he was clearly tired after dinner and meds as he stayed awake all afternoon. He said he would take his shower in the morning. So instead of a shower, I helped him with a sponge bath, no shampoo, followed by his series of topical ointments. He was ready to sleep, and I think he may have slept the whole night through. I checked around 2 A.M. and he was asleep.

Saturday morning, he was up before 7 A.M. and came out to the kitchen, happy to have his usual cup of black coffee in his usual chair while he looked at the sports and weather pages of the paper that we saved for him. But as for the shower, he said he always takes showers at night. I had a hunch he would do this, forgetting his promise to bathe this morning. So, I insisted he keep to his word in the evening, and we would definitely have a shower then. Promise.

Most of the morning he read the newspaper and we played card games (Match, Go Fish). In Match, one turns over pairs of cards in order to make a match. One must keep in mind, short-term, where the specific cards are. His ability to do this waxed and waned within the course of a single game. Sometimes he remembered well; other times, he couldn't seem to remember what was just turned over. His attention wandered, and he needed to be brought back to the game.

Two things stand out. First, Sunday morning around 4 A.M., I heard Pete moaning in his room. When I went to check, he was sitting up in bed backward, facing the head of the bed and looking toward his pillow, talking to himself or someone. I couldn't quite tell which. He said he couldn't sleep. He told me one of the puppets, named Mary, would not let him sleep. I lay down beside him to comfort him. Eventually he drifted off.

The second thing was while eating lunch, he stopped eating (rare!) and became silent and withdrawn. He just sat there, blank expression. When I tried to establish eye contact while touching him gently, he did not respond at all. Nothing. After quite some time, he came out of whatever mental state he had been in. I drove him back Sunday afternoon. He was very tired.

HOW I BEGAN AUTOMATIC WRITING

Decades earlier, when I was still living in California, I had worked with a past-life hypnotist and discovered I was a good hypnotic subject. I wondered now whether hypnotic trance might be a fruitful way to tap into some fertile source for writing poetry. I decided to experiment. There was no way for me to have known at that time how my automatic writing would take the significant and different course that it did in the years to come.

The history of automatic writing, in one form or another, includes the spirit writing from a thousand years ago in Song Dynasty China, to nineteenth-century spiritualism in this country, to the surrealist poets in early twentieth-century France, such as André Breton, who were influenced by Freud's ideas of the subconscious mind. They experimented with automatic writing to bypass the conscious mind and open up what might be found subconsciously. William Butler Yeats and his wife, George, in Ireland also engaged in extensive automatic script, some of which was the basis for his book, *A Vision,* and many of his later poems. There have been numerous studies and experiments to understand how it happens.

When I started, I used recordings that provided inductions into hypnotic trance. Later, without the benefit of a recording, I could put myself into a trance. I would begin writing sessions with a prayer or invocation and allow myself to enter a hypnotic trance state. With a pencil in hand and a pad of yellow legal paper, I would focus on my breathing and let my right arm write on its own. At first, my purpose for this process was to generate poems.

I did not stop to question the words that showed up on the paper, no matter how nonsensical they might seem to me. I wasn't exactly hearing the words, but my hand was writing them, and while writing, I was sometimes aware of the sound of the words in my mind. Once I was past my initial invocation and my stating any particular concerns, I made no conscious effort to influence what showed up on the page. The words appeared spontaneously. It took years to establish a productive routine for these automatic writing sessions. The trick was to drop deep enough into a trance to bypass my critical conscious mind but not so deep as to fall asleep.

Little by little, I became more adept at putting myself into such a trance—relinquishing control and yet still managing to write. I was skeptical about how it all worked and where the words were coming from. Despite my doubts, though, I continued the automatic writing practice.

The results were a meaningless jumble at first. Eventually, what showed up on the page was material I could craft into poems. Then a most startling thing happened. What also began to show up on my pages were the words of dead people—people that I had known—my mother, my father, and others. I was intrigued by this strange development. I didn't understand how it was happening, but these were people I had known, and their words were familiar.

Whenever I began a trance-writing session, I never knew what or who would show up on the page, even if I had asked for a particular person when I began. Eventually, the poetry part gave way to the more fascinating practice of conversing with the dead: first those whom I had known and then with other entities in the world of spirit.

After some time, the voice of an American poet, now deceased, showed up on the page. He volunteered to be a gatekeeper, opening the door to those in the spirit world who wished to speak and guarding against any ill-intentioned spirits. As he was a famous poet when he was living, he requested that I call him by the nickname Putty instead of his real name so I would not be distracted by his former life.

Even now, after years of this trance-writing practice, it is never clear to me whose voice might show up on the page. Sometimes I begin a session by asking a specific question or by calling for a particular person or spirit who may or may not respond. Other times I begin a session ready to hear from anyone about anything. In the trance conversations here, the dates before each section are the dates when the sessions were conducted. So as to avoid repetition, not every session here includes the full opening prayer or any particular focus for that session. Also, Putty, the gatekeeper whose voice shows up at every session after my opening prayer and requests, is not included in every session.

It is important to note that the dialogue, *all* the dialogue, is the actual word-for-word dialogue from the sessions. I have not added words or changed words although I have deleted repetitive material. The supplementary prose, in italics, is intended to provide some explanatory context. These comments were not part of the original trance conversations but added later.

The voices in the conversations that follow here began in March 2013, a few years after the diagnosis of Pete's Alzheimer's. I had heard that people with dementia were sometimes capable of communicating in other ways when normal speech deteriorated. I wondered whether, somehow, I could converse with my brother by means of the automatic trance writing. I had no idea how it might help, or if it would help at all, but I tried. I called on Pete, and, to my surprise and delight, he answered, but reluctantly, at first. Other than my own voice and Pete's, the voices are from the world of spirit, including family members who are deceased and others. When, in time, Pete lost the ability to speak or understand others' speech, he became more willing to converse in this unusual way. He seemed able, even eager, to communicate through the automatic writing when he was asleep; although, when awake, he couldn't say much and did not remember the nighttime conversations.

Eventually Pete emerged as part of Bigger Pete, who also speaks.

MARCH 25, 2013

Elizabeth: The arm is ready to move on its own. I put my hand in service. What does it write? Pete or Mom? I dedicate my intention here to Pete.

Elizabeth: Pete, is some part of you here?

Pete: Sis, I don't want to do this.

Elizabeth: Okay, never mind. Mom, are you there?

Mom: Yes, hello, dear. About Peter, he has had a long time in his isolation. I did what I could. It was hard to be his mother. But there were moments of joy and I learned so much from him and because of him. What are you to do now? You cannot know his mind. You cannot solve or take away what he must endure. By your being kind, he learns kindness. He needs kindness now. He is angry.

> *The disease came on gradually, hardly noticeably. Some staff people where Pete lived did not believe Pete had Alzheimer's at first. Little by little, Pete was beginning to show the debilitating effects of the disease. I tried my best to explain to him what was happening, but understandably, he was frustrated and angry.*

He doesn't like his life now. He thinks it is wasted. But he is, at some level, starting to understand what his life means. Do what you can. You are important to him. He may or may not say that, but you are. I am very glad for all you've done. I was hoping you would. That's all I'll say for now.

APRIL 1, 2013

Elizabeth: What to do about anything? I dedicate this to all you, dear ones who have passed.

Unidentified spirits: Oh, we all want to reassure you who have your own struggles, but open your arms and open your hearts to Pete, who will be called soon to us here. He has had a hard life but has known joy too. Do not berate yourselves for what you do not do, cannot do. He knows your efforts. He sees your efforts. You have made this end of his life better than it might have been.

As for you, your sadness now is linked with him. It cannot be helped. Just do your routines, get sleep, take it easy. We are all speaking as of one voice. We can do that. You need not single out just one of us here.

Even though I was curious as to who or what they were, the unidentified spirits spoke as a group and declined to identify themselves individually or by name.

A P R I L   3 ,   2 0 1 3

Elizabeth: Not feeling good today.

Dad: Hello, Elizabeth. I never thought I could reach you like this. There is a frustration observing from here wishing to involve ourselves. I died too soon.

He died at fifty-seven years of age.

So much more I would have done. Your mother is here. You will come too, but I hope not for a long time. I don't have much to say except to say I'm proud of you, especially what you're doing now—poetry, taking care of Peter. Pete-Repeat, he never liked my calling him that. He was hard to bring into my view of myself. On that, your mother was better, far better.

You must take care of yourself. Bodies need care. That is all I would say, but do please call on me, if you like. It is strange for me too to have this connection and you don't believe it. I know that's true.

Even though I was skeptical that I could really be conversing with the dead, I continued the writing practice anyway. I would sit quietly where and when I would not be disturbed, usually at my desk or sitting in bed, most often in the evening. How the words show up on the pad remains a mystery, and after years of this practice, I can still be skeptical, so I still need to put that skepticism aside and continue.

Just act as if it's real. It isn't a lie. It is real. Take care and come back. Goodbye for now.

J U N E   2 9 ,   2 0 1 3

Elizabeth: What about Pete, anything I need to know?

Mom: Hello, sweetie. About Pete, you may think it strange that I could say this, but he's already living on borrowed time, as they say, longer than what they told us he'd live to.

In the 1920s, life expectancy for someone with Down syndrome was only nine years and, by the early 1970s, had risen to only thirty years old. Pete was born in 1956, so Mom may have been referring to the life expectancy statistic rather than Pete's recent diagnosis of Alzheimer's disease.

He will have troubles from here on in. He's in a good place. Let him stay as long as possible. If he has to move, he'll go into a slump—a big kind of slump.

From the time that Pete was ten years old, he lived at one or another home set up for those with disabilities. At this time, Pete lived in a group home with five other older men. His home was one of six such homes built in a circle with a connecting hall between them all. The facility had its own day program, a therapeutic swimming pool, a meeting room for family conferences and lectures, a physical therapy room, staff offices, and a central enclosed courtyard. There was an outdoor walkway that circled the facility where I often walked with Pete, first when he walked on his own and later when he used a wheelchair. Each man had his own room and bathroom and shared a common living room and dining room with the other five men. The staff took care of cooking, cleaning, and accompanying the residents to doctors' appointments. Pete's room was bright and cheery. The big window looked out on three birch trees on the lawn at the back of the facility. He had his Eagles football things on the walls and around the room. When Pete first moved in, he said it was the best place he had lived.

Yes, send him cards, call him, go visit. It may not look as if he even notices. Do it anyway.

At the beginning of the conversations here, when his dementia was somewhat new, Pete's voice came in only briefly and quite reluctantly. However, as his dementia worsened, his normal speech became more difficult. Increasingly, he had trouble understanding the words of others and even more trouble producing words of his own that others could understand. He became more isolated. As it became more difficult for us to carry on a normal conversation face-to-face, this alternative method of conversing through trance writing allowed us to speak with each other, which we could not do otherwise. It seemed that his dementia did not affect his ability to converse when he was asleep, and we conversed via trance writing.

O C T O B E R   1 9 ,   2 0 1 3

Elizabeth: Pete, if you're sleeping, can you send a message? Or anyone on anything?

Pete: Hello, Sis, yes, I can talk to you better this way. My mouth and my brain just aren't working well. I'm glad you care. This is rough for me and for you. I can see that. That's why I want out. Let the noisy ones talk. I'll bow out and let them. I'm not always so angry as you think I might be. Sometimes I think this is what I deserve, that I had it coming. The next time around, I'll try better to be kinder.

I wasn't sure what he meant by "next time around." I was guessing he meant another life, but neither he nor I had spoken of other lives, whether past or future. Nor had we ever mentioned reincarnation. So, his words were surprising.

Come ask me again. I can talk to you this way. Thank you, Sis. I hug you.

Elizabeth: I am open to any spirit guides of any sort or deceased people or living people, anyone or anything that wishes to tell me what I need to know now.

Unidentified spirits: This is a group speaking. You need not know names. We have your best interests in mind, at heart, at present. Write our words.

Bless this day. It is a good one. We bless you in it. You are a good one. We take note of your doings, your thinkings, your wishes, your desires, your anxieties, your fears. We're here to guide you, to tell you what you need to hear.

About your brother, yes, you worry, but he needs you now. He relies on you more and more. Follow his lead but think through his requests. He does not always know the best for himself. He will talk later, but we want to say also don't wear yourself out. He can drain you. You know this is so. You sense the pull.

I was certainly feeling the pull in more ways than one. Physically, when Pete could still walk and we walked together, he would hold on tight to my arm, and because he was unsteady, he pulled hard on me. Emotionally too, witnessing his decline was draining for me. When leaving him after a visit, I would often sit in my car by myself, crying in sadness as I thought about Pete's struggles. Then I would collect myself before starting my long drive home.

Take care of him but take care of yourself. Your body is aging whether you like it or not. So is your brother's. So have some humor around that. That it's not always fun but it has its good points. Here is your brother.

Pete: I am here. I cannot talk well. I try, try again, but the words, they don't come. Thank you, Sis, for looking out for me. Thanks for the signs.

I had made door signs for Pete's room in the group home. One sign said, "You are welcome. Come in." The other sign said, "Not now. Come back later." These signs were for the puppets that Pete said he had been seeing but that no one else saw. Mostly the puppets were benign, but occasionally the puppets made noise and bothered him. The door signs were for Pete to use on those occasions when the puppets disturbed him. The signs had loops of string so that Pete could easily hang the signs on his doorknob or stand them up on his bedside table. I was hoping the signs might give Pete a degree of control over any unwelcome visitors.

I like that you listen to me. You're what I have left. My mother is gone. My father is gone. Soon I will be gone, maybe with them. Now I am here. You are here too. Bro and Sis. Do not be afraid if I decide to leave. That time's getting close. I may not stay until the last minute. I have learned many things. I did some things wrong. I do not want to do the wrong things. I'm getting tired. I want to enjoy a few more days, but do not be surprised if I leave soon. I mean leave for good.

You have been a good sister. You do your best. I can see that. I can say that. Not now because it's hard to talk. So very hard. How did this happen? Everything is so hard.

I'd like to leave when I am sleeping, go quietly, find my mother, my father where they are now. They were good to me, especially my mother. I don't have anything else to say now except I love you, Sis, and thank you for everything. I give you a hug. Goodbye, goodbye, goodbye, goodbye, goodbye.

DECEMBER 12, 2013

Elizabeth: I'm open to hearing from anyone—but Daddy, what an appearance!

I had had a dream of my father.

Dad: Hello, yes, this is your father.

Elizabeth: You looked so good, so very good in your yellow sweater. You looked great, sexy, if a daughter can say so.

Dad (laughing): Do you know what fun it is to hear you say that—about the looking good and sexy part? Marvelous. I'm so proud of you. I'm sorry I left so soon. You have much to do still in your life. I can say a bit more about why I am proud of you—your devotion to your writing, your hard work on it. It will pay off. Yes, you will see, perhaps even more notice than you want or think you deserve.

I'm also proud that you look out for Pete. He relies on you, especially now. I never really got over the shock of his birth. Your mother was better. Despite our troubles, I give her big credit for her support of him—and now you.

> *Mom was a tireless advocate for Pete. She sought out the best care she could find for him, took him on international trips with her, and, in so many imaginative ways, helped him to become his very best self.*

I'll back away but remember how proud I am, very proud.

Elizabeth: Thank you, Dad.

***

DECEMBER 23, 2013

Elizabeth: Pete, is there anything you can or want to tell me, Bro, or is this too strange? I'm feeling immensely sad this morning. The hand wishes to write. Whose voice?

Pete: Sis, I am here. Yes, strange. Maybe I can talk better this way. Sis, I am scared.

> *From time to time, when Pete was awake, I saw his face when he was scared. As he declined, the scared face became less frequent. Then he looked either more resigned or not seemingly present at all.*

I don't know what will happen, what will happen to me. Help me, Sis.

Elizabeth: I am here, Bro.

Pete: Stay near to me. Hold me. I think I am going somewhere. I don't know where. Sis?

Elizabeth: Yes?

Pete: Sis, please, take care of me.

Elizabeth: I'll do whatever I can. You do what you can. It may be hard. Are there things you want me to know?

Pete: I don't know, Sis. I don't know. Just stay near and remember me. Let me talk to you, if I can. Talk to me, Sis. I am scared. I don't know what will happen. I want someone to take care of me. I want someone to hold me, to keep me. That's all.

Elizabeth: Is it okay to talk like this?

Pete: Yes, maybe I can do this. Goodbye. That's all, Sis.

Pete called me "Sis" because he never had an easy time pronouncing my long name of Elizabeth. Sometimes, he would also call me "Teach" as a nickname.

MARCH 23, 2014

Elizabeth: Help with Pete?

Mom: Hello, my dear. You ask about Pete. About his eyes, think what to tell him, but hold off as long as you can for the surgery—summer at least—when you have more time, travel is easier. Yes, definitely talk to him about it but not too much. In this case, less is better. Take time to see if he understands. I send my love to you and through you to him.

Pete had cataracts. Pete's eye doctor showed me how to look through his lens instrument so I could see cataracts in Pete's eyes. The doctor explained the available options, including surgery. However, operating for cataracts had to be postponed because Pete wouldn't understand or do what was required for him to recover, such as wearing eye patches. Also, a hearing test resulted in his being prescribed a hearing aid. He didn't like the hearing aid. One day on a trip to a park, he managed to leave the hearing aid behind somewhere that no one else could manage to find it. That was the end of the hearing aid.

MAY 7, 2014

Elizabeth: I'm open to one and all, ready to write—Mom, others.

<hr>

Mom: Hello, dear. I am here and happy to say something to you. Learn all you can. I don't think you'll have a problem with Alzheimer's, at least not for a long time. You have too much protecting you, and you have so much work to do. If you are thinking about talking seriously to Pete—do so. He'll understand more than you suspect. There is no hurry.

Oh, about the incident when he left you last time. Not a problem. He needed that, very much needed that. Yes, you treated him like a child, but he was acting like a child.

Pete had been visiting us for some days and he didn't want to leave our house to go back to his group home. He refused to get in the car when it was time for me to drive him back. Because my husband and I were planning to travel the next day, Pete couldn't stay longer with us at that time, so my husband and I had to pick him up and put him in the car to drive him back to his place. It bothered me enormously that I had to do that.

He respects you for your insistence even though he needed very much to save face. One thing you can do though is be clear about times—when you will come for him, when he will be leaving.

MARCH 15, 2016
(TWO YEARS LATER)

The previous two years had been busier than usual for me as I was completing an MFA degree in poetry (via distance education so I wouldn't be geographically far from Pete). While Pete continued to decline, the rate of his decline up to this point seemed somewhat gradual, but now it seemed to be accelerating.

Mom: Hello, my dear. I want to say something that will sound strange but I'm wanting to be able to see Peter. I mean here, where I am. It's not up to me but I think I'm not alone. It may be coming close to the end of his time on Earth. I know you have prepared for this, but it will be demanding for you when the time comes.

And this writing you're doing, that I hope you will publish, will make people aware death is not such a strange thing and that something goes on. That does not negate mourning. People loved are missed. But for now, let me just cheer you on with all you do.

O C T O B E R   2 3 ,   2 0 1 6

Elizabeth: I am ready to write in the best interests of all in the spirit of Divine Love.

Mom: Hello, dear. I am more "into" this than many others here. They would speak if they knew they could be heard. Still, they send love and whatever they can. Can you believe there is even some jealousy that I can speak with you? Well, yes, we don't change miraculously when we pass on, but we certainly can reflect on the lives we have lived.

Mine should have been happier for all that it was, but I had a cloud and not always acknowledged. I took the medicine route to deal with depression. Pete relies on sleep. He is much with me now. At some point he'll come over in full.

Pete did take medication for depression. Depression is not a part of the intrinsic condition of Down syndrome, but it is a frequently diagnosed mental challenge for those with Down syndrome. For Pete, like some others with Down syndrome, he was sensitive to changes in his environment, but his response to change was sometimes delayed because any loss, such as with grief, took some time to register as a permanent change. Pete was very close to Mom, and when Mom passed away, Pete seemed to have a deep and long period of depression. He didn't want to go to the Day Program, choosing instead to sleep in his room.

* * *

JANUARY 1, 2017

Mom: Hello, my dear. About Pete, he is indeed aging. In some ways, he is getting tired—soul-tired of the life he is in. He has the habit of his charming self.

Pete did have a charming manner of using small gestures and pet phrases in an affectionate way, and, by so doing, he didn't have to talk as much or perhaps think about what would be appropriate that he could manage to say in a conversation. For example, he might ask me, "How's Teach?" and then he could relax and just listen to whatever I might answer. Or "Good idea, Sis," without further elaboration. He repeated his stock phrases so very often that it could sometimes be annoying until we remembered it probably made things easier for him. And we found ourselves using those handy comments of his ourselves.

He cannot stop the decline of his body. He will be ready soon to leave. He may not have learned all that he might, but his interest and drive (in his soul, I mean) are hampered by his physical obstacles. He will not want to press further after a while.

Pete was experiencing more medical problems. He was having a harder time moving around and relied on a walker and occasionally a wheelchair. His hearing and seeing were getting worse. He had dark moods more often.

Prepare for his going. You may be surprised the effect it will have on you—and surprised at the effect he has had on others. Continue to do your sisterly care, which has been enormous, and he has depended on. When it is time for him to leave, you should feel satisfied that you've done enough. As I've said before, contribute as you've been doing but never at detriment to yourself, please. And when the time comes, you will also see the realm that awaits you but <u>not for a long time</u> (underline that!).

At the beginning of each year, I would buy a desk calendar that had large spaces for each day. Sitting with Pete, I would enter the upcoming dates of interest to him. Increasingly, these events were doctors' appointments. I would write in what the appointments were for and the doctors' names and then draw a picture to match, such as teeth for the dentist or a foot for the podiatrist. Pete was amused at my pitiful attempts at drawing. I was never able to come up with a suitable drawing for his neurologist.

APRIL 25, 2017

Mom: Hello, my dear. Pete is indeed failing. He is losing interest in this life of his. At some level, he sees he has done all he could or rather all he is willing to do, or struggle to do. You are a comfort to him. You are what ties him to what is familiar, what is family. You will have to figure how to proceed, but his dark spells will increase in length and frequency. His bodily functions will start to function less well. You three should consider his options now.

Before she passed away, our mother had arranged that we three siblings of Pete should also serve as his legal guardians and make whatever decisions needed to be made for his care. For the most part, we were able to agree on such decisions when they pertained to Pete's well-being.

No, don't have him live with you. That is not your work. He may need to move, or he may need extra help. He does make efforts but is tired now of doing so. He wants relief. He'll want to sleep.

She was correct in that Pete began to sleep more and more. This allowed him to rest from his increasingly difficult life with Alzheimer's when he was awake.

A P R I L 2 6 , 2 0 1 7

Elizabeth: I open my hand and mind. I wonder, Bro, if you are quite asleep, if you can tell me what's happening with you. Are you wanting your own quiet time to think about things, to sort things out with the puppets or by yourself? If you cannot say, that is okay.

Pete alone saw the puppets. He heard them and spoke with them. They traveled with him. When I drove back and forth to his place, Pete would sit in the front passenger seat and speak with the puppets. Gradually, I was able to understand more details about Pete's puppets. He saw them as small beings on the floor by his feet. I was fascinated by the puppets. I asked Pete if he would convey messages back and forth to the puppets for me, but Pete didn't quite see the point in that. "Not make sense," he would say.

Putty: Hello. I am here at the gate, and all is well.

Putty, the nickname for a deceased American poet, served as my gatekeeper to the world of spirit. His voice didn't appear on the page until I was several years into this automatic writing practice. It wasn't as if I somehow heard him and then he appeared in the writing. Rather, like all the other voices, they first appeared to me on the page, unlike the process with mediums who, through clairvoyance or clairaudience, see or hear those in the spirit world (other than by doing automatic writing). At first, we spoke of poetry. Putty taught me poetry and gave me marvelous exercises to do. But even when not speaking of poetry, he continued to serve as a gatekeeper. Somehow, he would make sure that any voices that wished to speak from the world of spirit were well-intended.

Pete: Sis, I am fine. I just want to think and think by myself. I don't want to go out. Out is okay but I just want to be here in my room by myself. Sometimes the puppets come, sometimes there are many. I like to talk to them. They tell me things, nice things, where I might go next. I know there is nothing you can do now, Sis. Really, I'm fine.

I am not sad, just quiet and thinking. And they tell me things I can't really tell you. Sis, I am fine. Bed bug bite.

"Bed bug bite" was abbreviated from our years-long habitual telephone sign-off, especially at night: "Good night, sleep tight, don't let the bed bugs bite."

***

M A Y   2 ,   2 0 1 7

Elizabeth: I am ready to write. Dad, did you want to say something? Pete, are you sleeping?

Dad: Hello, Elizabeth. Yes, I would speak to you in this way I never imagined when I was living with you. When it is time for you to come here, you will experience the joy, the beauty, the bliss, but you have still so much to give. Do it. There are many, so many, who do support you.

I may come in your dream, yes. But whoever else is around, you are the one who can see and sense. You are the one who listens and writes. I know you can't imagine who would publish your work. Do not worry about that now. Just get it ready. This is most important.

Don't worry about Pete. Nothing you can do there. He is on his own path—difficult, yes, but it is his path, not yours. You do what you can and that is a lot. You may not see it, but I can see it from here. I am not alone. I have been requested to send you this message of encouragement and support. I would do so anyway. You know your age and your energy. It won't last forever. This is my message. Do you hear me, Elizabeth?

Elizabeth: Yes.

Dad: All right then. That's why I have come—to tell you this. Know that I am rooting for you.

Pete: Sis, hello, Sis. I am talking to you, but it is so hard to talk now. My talking's not working.

Elizabeth: Yes, Bro, I am seeing that. I am so sorry. Do you think it will get better?

Pete: Sis, I'm going down. I'm tired and I'm scared.

Elizabeth: Bro, I don't like that you are scared. Is that why you talk to the puppets? Do they help?

Pete: Yes, they tell me everything will be all right.

Elizabeth: I think so too. Everything will be all right.

Pete: I don't know, Sis. Maybe I will die or go away, or I don't know what.

Elizabeth: Bro, I believe strongly that whatever happens to you, everything will be all right.

Wherever you go, whatever you do, everything will be okay. You will be happy.

Pete: Thanks, Sis. Thanks, Sis.

MAY 11, 2017

Putty: Hello, my dear young poet. There are several here who wish to speak. I open the gate.

Elizabeth: Thank you, Putty.

Mom: Hello, dear. I do hang around because I want to encourage and be available as things with Pete happen. He does not need to go through a long-drawn-out decline. He can come any time. There is no fault in your letting him know that. You can simply say something like: Bro, when you are ready, when you are tired and have had enough of this life, you can go on. It is okay. It will be okay for everyone, or at least for me. I will miss you, but I believe there is something else better for you after this life. We have had good lives as brother and sister. I have learned much from you, and I am glad you have been my brother. I do not want to see you have a hard time or have more troubles with your body than you already have. You have been more patient than I would have been. It may be possible for you and me to talk even when no longer alive, whether I go first or you do. I am not suggesting at all that you go now. I am only saying, go when you are ready and don't worry about me.

Elizabeth: Mom, I guess I took over writing that myself.

Mom: Yes, maybe you did. And it is good what you wrote, and Pete will understand at some level. You <u>will</u> miss him. But I think you well realize he has his own path. Thank you for listening, taking it to heart.

When Pete was losing language and we couldn't talk face-to-face, in my distress, I wrote this poem:

WHEN WORDS DESERT YOU

How do I love you now when you have changed so?
Where is my brother, sweet and gentle? Vanished!
Where is that tree whose pith runs strong and steadfast?
Felled in the forest.

You cannot give an answer. Words desert you.
I cannot find you. Can you find yourself now?
Home of your self slams shut its doors. You're homeless.
Where are you hiding?

When I look in your eyes, I see no flicker.
When I say something, anything, you are elsewhere.
Where do you go when this world gets too heavy?
Somewhere delightful?

You have your puppets. Only you can see them.
Can they protect you, cheer you, help you, keep you?
Brother, I miss you, wish you easier travels.
Yes, I still love you.

CHAPTER TWO

THINKING ABOUT WHAT
COMES NEXT

~~~~~~~~~~~~~~~~~~~~~~~~~~~~~~~~~~~~~~

M A Y   1 6 ,   2 0 1 7

Mom: Hello, dear. When Pete joins me here, we will have much to deal
with, given his life, his previous lives, and so forth. No, I won't say
more about that now. I expect you will hear from him when he does
come here. For now, thanks, as you accompany him down his path.

Pete: Sis?

Elizabeth: Yes, I am here, Bro.

Pete: Sis, I am scared. It seems my life is beginning to end.

Elizabeth: Yes, Bro, I would be scared too, but I don't think we need to
be scared. I believe there is more when we die, maybe much better
because I think it is without these bodies of ours that can give us
trouble. Are your puppets helping you be less scared?

Pete: Yes, Sis.

Elizabeth: That's good. You can tell me about the puppets or anything
else you want to.

> *Once, when I asked Pete to tell me more about the puppets, he
> simply said, "Sis, **not** the Muppets!" but he didn't elaborate. I was
> so very curious about the puppets, but although Pete could see them,
> they remained a mystery to me.*

Pete: Okay, Sis, but words are hard.

Elizabeth: Yeah, I know. Anyway, I am planning to come see you tomorrow. So, sleep tight.

Wake up. Go to Day Program, have a good day tomorrow.

In the group of group homes where Pete lived, the weekday Day Program included occasional trips to sporting events, museums, bookstores, and so forth. Sometimes Pete chose to sleep rather than to go. At this point, because his decline with Alzheimer's had been so gradual, I hadn't yet realized how much more difficult everything was getting for Pete as he declined with Alzheimer's.

Why, Bro, do you not go to Day Program?

Pete: Sis, I don't know. It is such an effort. It's easier to sleep and I feel better after.

Elizabeth: Oh, okay, Bro. Well, see you tomorrow.

A U G U S T   1 7 ,   2 0 1 7

Elizabeth: Good morning, all. I am writing to ask about Pete and his medical situation.

Unidentified voices: We are gathered for you, dear daughter of Earth. We come screaming across miles in a flash, but miles mean nothing to us. We can say something about your brother. Do what you can. Most of all, he will appreciate your presence. Plan to be with him. He will be glad for it, learn from it too. And do <u>not</u> fault yourself for whatever happens. You just play your role which you've played so well—sister and guardian and now also comforter. Does this all comfort you?

Elizabeth: Yes.

Unidentified voices: Well then know you can always count on us, dear daughter of Earth.

S E P T E M B E R   2 4 ,   2 0 1 7

Elizabeth: I am ready and willing and I hope able to hear from anyone about anything.

Unidentified spirits: Hello, Elizabeth. Do not trouble yourself about who is speaking. We come to encourage your current efforts. Before long, your brother will be called to us here. He has done all he can with his life there, as he knows it. He is tapping into what's next for him, how to make sense of the life he is finishing. He is grateful to you and recognizes your commitment.

And he will assist <u>you</u> when he moves on, but there's no need to say more.

O C T O B E R 1 , 2 0 1 7

Elizabeth: I am ready to receive whatever wisdom is available to my hand. About Pete?

Mom: Hello, dear, love to you and to Pete. His life's not been easy, but he is almost ready to leave it. It is his decision. It may be what seems a flash decision, but he has been mulling many things for a while.

N O V E M B E R 1 8 , 2 0 1 8

Mom: Hello, dear. I am glad you'll see Pete on Thanksgiving. If you go to him, it's less difficult.

When Pete visited us for Thanksgiving, one of the things he always seemed to like was that I would print out a fancy menu of all the food I had prepared for our dinner. He would keep the menu by his plate and make sure I presented each item as listed. Later, when it was time for me to drive him back, he would be sure to pack the menu, as a souvenir of sorts, in his suitcase.

At dinner, whether Thanksgiving or any other meal, Pete enjoyed playing a game of food groups in which we, in turn, would name a food group, like vegetables, and then each, in turn, would have to name a vegetable until someone couldn't think of any more vegetables. That's when the game got goofy, and Pete, especially, would offer crazy items like "asparagus ice cream" or "potato chip beans" just so he wouldn't end up the loser.

By now, we had made all the physical accommodations for his visits—wheelchair ramps, bathroom equipment—that were possible in our old house. So, as his physical needs increased, his coming to us had to change to our going to him instead for safety reasons.

If I say give him a hug for me, he may not understand but who knows. He has been tapping more into his own soul these days—not that you'd see it, but I do.

Elizabeth: Really? Wow.

MARCH 24, 2019

Elizabeth: I ask for whatever I need or would want to know about Pete, what is coming.

Putty: Hello, my dear. About your brother: he is readying himself to let go of life. He does like to see you, be with you. No need to talk, much as you like to chatter. So, go easy. Let him lead any conversation. He knows you are there, that you care.

Little by little, I learned that it isn't important—in fact, it can be downright inconsiderate—to chatter on and on with someone with Alzheimer's disease. For that someone to keep up a conversation can be almost impossible. Just being with someone quietly is still being with them. In fact, I noticed that Pete had been gravitating to those staff people who were quieter, or at least quieter when around him.

MAY 2, 2019

Elizabeth: I am ready to receive anything I should know about Pete—his seizure hospitalization, new meds.

Pete had been hospitalized because of seizures. Another medication was added to the many he was taking. He was already taking

medicines for depression, osteoporosis, urinary tract infections,
allergies, incontinence, osteoarthritis, foot fungus, dementia, and
others. Whenever a new medication was suggested, I requested a
review of what he was already taking, not just to avoid possible bad
drug interactions but to keep the chemical soup in his body as much
to a minimum as possible. Luckily, Pete never objected to taking
his medications, probably because we put the bad-tasting ones in
applesauce before he took them.

Mom: Hello, dear. Yes, Pete is nearly at the end of his life. I have said this before, but remember, I speak from where time doesn't happen. He is hanging on because it is what he knows. You can reassure him, not in spoken words, which his brain has a hard time with, but speak to him like this—in spirit, in your dreams, in your prayers. He knows he owes you much for all your care. He cannot tell you in words, but he has, hasn't he? When he says, "Thank you," it is a big one, and his saying thank you is important for him to do.

J U N E   1 0 ,   2 0 1 9

Elizabeth: I need help. I feel in a tangle.

Unidentified spirits: Dear, dear, Elizabeth: about your brother, he is getting ready to leave, to come home. He cannot tell you this in words. Allow him to go when he is ready.

Elizabeth: Dear Pete, this is your sister Elizabeth speaking to you. I know you are getting ready to leave this life. I know you are afraid, not a lot but a little. But I see you are tired and ready to go home, and home is with Mom, with Dad, with the angels where you are your best and most wonderful self. I have been able to see a little bit of what comes next when you leave this life.

You will be glad to be there.

I had a near-death experience during the years I lived in West
Africa. I had been teaching preparation for childbirth classes in

a hospital in Accra, having trained to do that with the National Childbirth Trust in England. I contracted malaria and went into a coma but survived. I didn't know about near-death experiences until I had that one myself, but one effect was that it substantially reduced my fear of death. Another effect was that I became more curious about a number of things that I would consider mysteries, and probably, that experience made me more amenable to such things as past-life regressions and automatic writing.

Of course, I will miss you. I have learned much from you—about patience, acceptance, trust, and simple, kind, human connection.

You are my brother. I have tried to be a good sister. I will miss you. Many will, but if you need my permission to leave this life, you have my permission. Go when you are ready to leave your body that is not working so well and be your free and wonderful self.

It may be we can still talk in this way. I love you, Bro. I'll be listening and meanwhile watching out for you, for your life still ahead. So, hugs, dear Bro, lots of hugs, lots of love.

Goodbye for now.

J U N E 1 7 , 2 0 1 9

Elizabeth: I open my heart. Pete, if you are asleep and feel like talking, I am listening.

Putty: Hello, dear one. You are loyal, faithful to this project, to those you care for with so little reward.

> *Putty's comment about caring "with so little reward" resonated with me. I was becoming familiar with a number of caregivers of people with Alzheimer's. One bit of advice that was circulated frequently was to be prepared for much work and heartache for many years but with little reward.*

Mom: Hello, dear. I hope you don't mind. I have become a part of your circle of support over here, and when you ask for Pete, of course I am interested. He is not in distress. He is going along on his path. He is happy to speak with you. He likes the familiar, especially now, as he is coming upon many new things.

By the way, he does thank you over and over. You are the steady thing in his life. He knows you are there, watching and caring. He has learned much from you—your kindness, your steady care, your being available. What he can say now, what he can do, will become less and less. His attention, when he can muster it, is on what's next and whether he has permission to finish this life.

Get your rest. You are tied in tight to what he's going through, and it is tiring. Well, that's enough from me for now.

Elizabeth: Thanks, Mom.

Unidentified spirits: Elizabeth, we call on you as you call on us. We know you wish to know who we are. If you can manage without knowing that, that would be better. You can think of us this way. There are many who support you—those who lived and passed on, those who've never lived, on Earth at least. There are angels, archangels, your own higher self. When someone like you is as faithful and caring, you have the attention, the help of many. We know you will make good use of it all.

Also, get rest. Part of the rest will be for the emotional toll on your body. Part of your rest allows for your listening in ways you cannot when you're awake. At those times, you join the circle of folks—elders—who share with you and your brother their help and support. So, rest is a good use of time. Do you understand?

Elizabeth: Yes, I think so, and I thank you.

J U N E 1 9 , 2 0 1 9

Elizabeth: With open heart, ready hand, I ask if I might speak with Pete if he is so inclined.

Pete: Oh, hi, Sis. Yes, I am here. It is easier to sleep.

Elizabeth: I think I understand. Sometimes the awake things just get too hard. What can I do to make things less hard?

Pete: You are fine. Just keep doing whatever you do. I am tired, need to rest, not just from this day. I need to rest from all of this life. It is too hard to do everything. Come see me sometimes. I may not talk but I'm glad you're here.

Elizabeth: Okay, I'll come Thursday to see you. Do you want me to bring you anything?

Pete: No, Sis, just come and see me. We can hug, smile, then say good-night, bed bug bite.

J U N E   2 3 ,   2 0 1 9

Elizabeth: I am here with open heart, ready hand for anyone's words.

Aunt Elizabeth: Hello, dear Elizabeth.

> *Aunt Elizabeth was Mom's sister, my aunt and namesake. I grew especially close to her when I was at college in Berkeley, California, and she lived nearby in Lafayette. She believed that when people died, that was the end, that there was no afterlife. Here, she is speaking from the afterlife.*

It has been a grand readjustment to what I am experiencing now, especially since I had no clue about all this before. But it is glorious, I assure you. You can pass on such assurances to brother Pete.

Your mother, energetically as always, is watching him, ready to welcome him when he joins us here. His path is unique. He is not served by living much longer now. He has learned much. I can say that. And I know you have learned much from him. That is good news you should share with many who might not see the gifts he can give. Do say so whenever you can. And tell him too. His coming here occupies him now. He is tying up loose ends there even if he could not at all say that to anyone now.

From what I can gather, I would not be surprised if he will be in touch with you when he's here. It may take some time, as it has for me, but he is beholden to you, his sister. But do carry on with your own work and life. My dear, my dear namesake, you have so much more good living ahead. Do not squander it by burning yourself out. You would be surprised how many are cheering you on, including me. I am so proud of you. I admire you immensely.

Elizabeth: Thank you, Aunt Elizabeth.

Aunt Elizabeth: I send my love, cloudfuls of love.

A U G U S T   7 ,   2 0 1 9

Elizabeth: I am ready, my heart open, to write whatever those in spirit wish to say.

Unidentified spirits: Hello, Elizabeth. Yes, those of us do wish to speak. We wish to support you in this work of yours and commend you for recognizing this is your work now. It is good you are giving up your poetry work.

After retiring from college teaching, I rediscovered my love of poetry. I started writing and publishing poetry and went back to school for a master's degree in poetry. After ten years or so of poetry, I realized my focus was shifting away from writing poetry to writing nonfiction works of a more spiritual nature, so I was indeed giving up poetry.

About your brother, yes, it's close to time for him to pass on. He is okay more and more with the thought of his own passing. Reassure him that he's doing well, that he is on his right path, that many will miss him when he decides he will leave. But so many will remember him fondly. But then, be prepared. He will want to speak with you. When he does pass on, he will open up to you new wisdom. You do have choices. You have chosen to see him through. You have been a true sister, and he wishes, when he can, to acknowledge that and show you his gratitude. Now that is all on that.

Elizabeth: Thank you.

Unidentified spirits: We know you wish to know who we are. You want to know names. Why do you need them? You need our messages. Perhaps the names are some grasping for proof. We know you want that, but you do not need it. You have developed trust in our existence, our willingness, even eagerness to help you along.

Because of my skepticism, one of the biggest challenges for me all along was developing trust in the communications coming from the world of spirit, the other side of life.

A U G U S T   8 ,   2 0 1 9

Elizabeth: I come with open heart and ready hand. I wonder if you are asleep, Pete, and could talk with me—tell me how you are doing.

Pete: Hello, Sis. Thank you for calling me. I am happy to see you, to hear you. I know I am changing, not saying much when you come to see me.

Indeed, Pete was disappearing into himself. I could sit with him quietly, but he often seemed more absent than present.

My body is having hard times. Sometimes it hurts, so I disappear and let it be. Every little thing is so difficult. I am glad for the help. And I thank you, Sis. I know you are watching out for me. You see I can talk when I can do it like this. Otherwise, it is too easy to get confused. Talk all around me. What are they saying? Hugs are nice. Your hugs are nice, Sis.

Elizabeth: I'm falling asleep.

Pete: Go to sleep, Sis. I am sleeping too. Let's say goodnight.

In the beginning, I would conduct these conversations while in a hypnotic trance in my house in Pennsylvania and when I guessed Pete would be asleep in his home in New Jersey. So, it was better to conduct the sessions at night when Pete would most likely be asleep. As a result, an ongoing challenge for me at night was staying in trance without falling asleep. As Pete declined, he slept more during the day, so sometimes I could converse with him in the daytime and then I could stay awake more easily.

A U G U S T 9 , 2 0 1 9

Elizabeth: I open my heart and ready my hand to write words of any-one—Pete, if he is able.

Pete: Hi, Sis. Here I am. Thank you for talking with me, caring for me. I cannot tell you easily in words, but I can tell you like this. So many things are happening, new things I don't understand and then some-times there is nothing at all. Sometimes I am scared, sometimes just quiet. Sometimes I am curious, sometimes just tired. I feel someone is ready to hug me, is somewhere nearby, but I can't see who it is. Is it you, Sis? I don't know.

Elizabeth: Bro, I don't know either. If you and I can talk like this, it is good. We are not speaking. We are not near each other, but somehow your self is talking to my self and I am writing down the words we are thinking or dreaming. And that is okay. I like it. Do you?

Pete: Yeah, Sis. It isn't easy to talk. My thinking is not easy, but I can do this. Something of me is talking to you. I hear other voices some-times too. I think I hear Mom. She says she loves me.

It is strange but not scary. Can you understand, Sis?

Elizabeth: Yes, Bro, I think so.

Pete: Thank you, Sis. I am lucky. I have had a good life. People have cared for me even when I can't care for myself. But I think my life is almost over. I don't really know, but it feels like that.

Is that okay?

Elizabeth: Yes, I think it's okay. I am glad that you have had a good life. I think I have too, but I don't think my life's almost over. I want to live some more years, do more writing and stuff. But sometime my life will be over. That happens to everyone. We don't live in our bodies forever, but I think we can still live, just not in our bodies.

Pete: How, Sis?

Elizabeth: I can't really say, Bro. It is what I believe. There is a soul or spirit—our best, most special self—that can live on without a body. What do you think?

Pete: I don't know, Sis. I know that my body has its own troubles, but some part of me hardly notices that. My back hurts sometimes, my face hurts sometimes. My hands and feet feel cold and funny. Sometimes they do not feel part of me. I look at my hand. I know it's my hand. It's attached to my arm, my arm to the rest of me. But there it is, and it can seem like it has its own life. Did I never tell you this?

Elizabeth: No, Bro, you never did. Maybe it was hard to explain, or maybe you thought I would not understand. But your telling is very good, Bro. Is there more that you wish to say to me now?

Pete: Not right now, but I like talking like this. I love you, Sis.

AUGUST 11, 2019

Elizabeth: I ask if I might continue the words with Pete.

Pete: Hello, Sis. I am here. I can speak. We have stops and starts but the love just goes on and on. My body is resting, my old, worn-out body. We do what we can when we can, and often it's not as much as we wish for. Our wishings pull us out way ahead of ourselves. I know all about that. I have learned to live with wishing for more than I could ever do. And now, even more, my body is doing its very best, but it gets harder and harder. I don't know what's next. Sometimes I am curious, sometimes I am scared. I think it's my body that's getting scared, afraid of its own ending, but mostly I'm curious of what's coming next. So, it's a matter of letting things be.

Elizabeth: Bro, you sound so wise. Your words are wonderful. I learn from you, Bro.

AUGUST 12, 2019

Elizabeth: In the wisdom of Divine Light and Love, I open my heart and ready my hand.

Dad: Hello, Elizabeth. Your mother and I are not enemies, although we divorced. You have a sense of the pressures we felt. Yes, Peter was one. Your mother went gung-ho, seeking the best. I was slow to realize it was not about me. Yes, I had a hard time, but also her whole gung-ho-ness was not always easy. She was ready to correct the whole world, me included. Well, that was then. This is now. We are not enemies. On different paths, yes, but we both love you all dearly and are so proud.

Elizabeth: You were a great father. I am so glad we can continue talking like this.

A U G U S T   2 4 ,   2 0 1 9

Elizabeth: My hand is ready to write. If Pete is wishing to talk, so am I.

Pete: Hello, Sis. I am glad when you talk with me like this.

Elizabeth: Yes, Bro, I am glad too. We can say whatever we like to each other this way. May I ask you questions?

Pete: Sure, go ahead, Sis.

Elizabeth: Can you tell me more about your puppets?

Pete: Yes, Sis. I know you like them. So do I. They are my friends. Some go with me when I go places. If I call them, they come, but they come on their own too. They talk to me but not regular talking, not like you and me talking. Their talk sounds like quiet, happy music, like water in a creek. I can't remember all their names, but the names are kind of funny.

A U G U S T   2 6 ,   2 0 1 9

Elizabeth: If Pete is asleep and therefore available, I would like to hear from him. Or anyone.

Pete: Hi, Sis. I am here.

Elizabeth: Pete, I started to talk last night, but I fell asleep. Sorry. Is there anything special you want to tell me or ask me now?

Pete: Yes, Sis, so many things. I like doing this, but how does it work?

Elizabeth: Pete, I can't explain it. People say when we talk like this, we are talking soul to soul.

Can you understand that?

Pete: I don't know. It's like a little hidden but important part of me is talking, not really as Pete.

That's just the name of my body.

Elizabeth: Yes, that sounds right. And I'm not really just Elizabeth. That's the name of my body now. Can you tell me more about who you are as you are talking to me now? Are you Pete or something else?

Pete: It's me but it's bigger than me, or maybe smaller than me. It's not easy to explain.

Elizabeth: Are you somewhere where you can see Mom or Dad?

Pete: Not right now, but sometimes I can see, especially Mom, and she's smiling and is glad to see me. She says I can come to where she is if I want to.

Elizabeth: Do you want to?

Pete: Yes, maybe. It's very nice and I like the way I am when I see her.

Elizabeth: Pete, I can only guess, but I think where Mom is is where we all go when we die. Not really die, but we leave our bodies behind and become something else. I think we become our true selves without any aches or pains. Does that make sense to you?

Pete: Yes, sort of. It's bright and kind and I like it. It's different.

Elizabeth: Well, Bro, if you decide you want to go there all the time, I think we can still talk like this together. At least I hope so.

Pete: Me too, Sis. Let's talk again.

AUGUST 27, 2019

Elizabeth: My heart is open, my hand ready to write words from anyone, maybe Pete.

Pete: Hello, Sis. I call you that now. It is in our bodies as brother and sister that we know each other, but you and I have lived before, known each other before, but I leave that at that for now. Pete is asleep—that is, my physical body is asleep, so I am free to travel here and there to talk with you.

> *The way Pete was speaking here, including about other shared lives, seemed strangely different to me—somehow more knowledgeable, wiser, well-spoken. Not quite like the Pete I knew.*

You can ask me questions if you wish. I'll try to answer if I can do so but for limited time. Do you have questions?

Elizabeth: Yes, oh so many. One is, does your physical mind and body have any knowledge or awareness of what you do when asleep?

Pete: Some knowledge, but most is lost when waking up. There's a residual tone that sometimes lingers but the gap is wide. My physical mind would get confused and also frustrated at not being able to connect the two or to tell what it's about. That is one reason I like this conversation. You probably have a hard time yourself putting what I say here now with who I am in my physical body and mind, which is on its last legs, so to speak.

> *I had a hard time making sense of what didn't sound like Pete. Pete didn't usually use words like "residual tone" or refer to his body in this distant way—"its last legs, so to speak."*

I am becoming resigned to those problems. It won't last much longer. And people are kind and take care of me. I am thankful for that. I try to be thankful, let them know if I can. Like you, Sis.

Being able to talk like this with you is wonderful, so very wonderful.

Elizabeth: Do you think it's okay if I talk to others about these conversations?

Pete: It is okay, yes, quite okay, but some will not understand so think about that. But yes, many will think when they see me that I am incapable of much, but you can see, I hope, that those incapacities are limited to the physical mind and body. So, it's a relief for me to sleep and to travel, to be my bigger, higher, whatever-you-want-to-call-it self.

And up to this point, I had not heard Pete mention a "bigger, higher" self.

It would be good for others to consider that something similar may be happening with others. If others would like to hear and consider these conversations, we wouldn't want to hoard them to ourselves, right?

I believe we can continue to "talk" even when I leave all the physical body behind. I'm almost ready for that but not quite yet. I am going to stop talking now, but let's talk again, anytime, anytime. I love you, Sis. Take care of your wonderful self.

AUGUST 29, 2019

Elizabeth: I thank in advance any who would speak, if possible, Pete.

Pete: Hello, Sis. Yes, I am here. This makes me feel good to talk with you. You have been a good sister and now we have this. Pete is asleep, his body and mind, my body and mind. I know you don't trust it, but I know you have learned how to do this anyway, even if you and I do not understand. And I know I will sound different from the brother you know or think you know.

But I will say this: You have always been able to see further than my most obvious limitations, and I'm glad for that. And I know my sometimes-strange ways annoy or upset you. But isn't that often in families or friends?

Do you want to ask me something? You always have questions!

Elizabeth: Do you have any suggestions for how I can learn to trust this process more?

Pete: I think you have already learned that. Just keep doing what you do, even with your doubts.

Elizabeth: How is it you sound so very wise? Aren't I making this, your words, up?

Pete: Well, that's the doubt speaking. I am sure it boggles the mind for you to believe I am your brother, Pete, but think of me and yourself as ever so much more than we think we know. Think of anyone as much more than what we see and hear usually. That's true of all of us, and isn't it marvelous?!

Pete's voice was definitely sounding different, wiser, more than the usual Pete I thought I knew.

A U G U S T   2 9 ,   2 0 1 9

Elizabeth: I am here, heart open, hand ready to write. Take my arm, guide it to write.

Pete: Hi, Sis—it's Pete or what you might call Bigger Pete.

Elizabeth: Are you okay? Your physical self went to the hospital this morning. Did you fall in the night?

Pete: Yes, Sis. I did. I wasn't fully awake. I don't know where I thought I was going. I'm okay, just not too good in the old body.

Pete got out of bed in the night, but the staff in his group home did not see him get up.

Elizabeth: And now, where are you? Who are you? What about your body?

Pete: Oh, so hard to explain. Not because of my mouth and brain not working but because it's hard to describe. I am no real place, but I am definitely here—what's important about me, what is truly me, is here. No aches, pains, hurts.

Elizabeth: Is it okay to talk like this? Or does it mess you up at all?

Pete: Yes, do talk like this. I like it very much. Maybe it will mess me up a little. I don't know how. Who can I really talk to? Especially now. People like smiles and gestures, but I feel very isolated, like I'm on an island by myself with a huge unswimmable ocean around me. I like that we can talk. Please, please continue.

Elizabeth: I feel I'm getting sleepy.

Pete: Well then, go to sleep. Maybe we can jump in each other's dreams. Want to try?

Elizabeth: Sure, let's.

Pete: Okay then, good night, sweet dreams.

────────── ∿∿∿∿∿ ──────────

AUGUST 30, 2019

Elizabeth: I am ready to write the words of any who would speak.

──◎

Pete: Hello, Sis. I am here. I am getting ready to leave. I have seen Mom. She is waiting for me,

I know. We have so much to do when we pass on. I am getting a little idea of it. It feels strange and yet like home, a wonderful home. Now, do you have all your usual questions?

Elizabeth: Oh yes, I wonder how you are, and I can be talking like this while you had something like an accident in your physical body.

> *In the night, Pete got out of bed and then fell in his room. When the night staff came into his room, they discovered his mouth was bleeding.*

They said you must have fallen in the night, bumped your head so it bled, and you knocked a tooth loose or out. Could all that have been happening while we were "talking"? I hope not. I like talking with you like this but not if it means you fall down and hurt yourself. What can you tell me?

Pete: Oh, Sis, sometimes my life feels so bumpy. I am not sure where I am—if I am awake or I am asleep. My eyes can be open—my physical eyes—but my mind is somewhere else. You know this. You have seen it. I cannot control it well. Something else is at work. It feels like traveling between two worlds—one familiar but difficult, the other beautiful but strange. I am trying to put the pieces together, but I feel confused sometimes, and I am not sure if I am in one world, the other, or somewhere between. That's why I feel good talking to you. You're like a guide or traveling companion who knows a little about both these worlds.

> *It did seem as if there were not only two worlds but two Petes. There was the Pete I knew who, aging with Down syndrome and now Alzheimer's, was becoming less verbal, less present when awake and*

then this Pete who seemed to speak so much more easily when his body was asleep.

And even if you don't know everything, you are willing to listen and hold my hand. Sometimes I feel happy, especially in that other world, sometimes confused, and sometimes just curious and trying to understand what is going on. Sis, I trust you completely.

Elizabeth: Take good care of your wonderful self.

S E P T E M B E R 1 , 2 0 1 9

Elizabeth: Here I am, hand ready to surrender to spirit, open to whoever would speak. Pete?

Pete: Hi, Sis—thank you for talking with me. I feel so in between. I think now about my life, what it means, what my life has been about, what happens next. Sometimes I feel lost, sometimes scared. I am glad when someone I know stays close to me, someone I can count on. Like you, Sis.

Elizabeth: Bro, you have many who stay close and support you, even if you cannot see them.

Pete: How do I know they are there?

Elizabeth: Trust, believe that they are. And sometimes, sometimes, you can feel the love.

Pete: Sis, where are you?

Elizabeth: I am in my house in Pennsylvania. You know my house, your room in our house, your favorite chair in the kitchen.

Pete's room was on the first floor of our house, which was good when he couldn't do stairs anymore. In the kitchen, he had his favorite chair next to the refrigerator. Eventually his wheelchair replaced that chair.

I am upstairs now and writing my words on a pad of yellow paper, and as I think of them, the words fly to you. I believe that you can receive them and that your words are coming back to me, the words you are thinking or dreaming. Does that make sense?

Pete: Yes, Sis. Thank you, Sis. It is good when I don't feel so good to know someone cares about me. Can I say something else?

Elizabeth: You can say whatever you wish to say.

Pete: I am going to have a good day today.

Elizabeth: I'm glad to hear that, Bro. I hope you have an excellent day today, wherever you are, wherever you go, whatever you do. Do you want to say goodbye for now?

Pete: Yeah, Sis. Goodbye for now.

S E P T E M B E R   2 ,   2 0 1 9

Elizabeth: My heart is open; hand is ready to write. Are you there, Bro? Want to talk?

Pete: Hello, Sis. My body is resting, but I can talk with you. I like to do this.

Elizabeth: Bro, you said you were thinking about what comes next after this life? Have you been thinking about that?

Pete: Yeah, Sis. I have. I think about it a lot.

Elizabeth: And what do you think?

Pete: Well, I think I can go where Mom is. It's nice there.

Elizabeth: That sounds good. You also said you were thinking about your life, that it has been good. Is that right?

Pete: Yeah, Sis. I have had a good life, but now it's hard. I get tired, confused, can't see well. I can't hear well. I forget where I am. And it's too hard to put the words together right. I can't walk well, can't get comfortable. That's why sleep is nice. I like to sleep. I don't have to talk or walk. I just take it easy. Remember, Sis?

Elizabeth: Yes. Walk, talk, relax, and take it easy.

> *This was one of Pete's all-time favorite expressions. Pete had a number of favorite expressions, many of which seemed to make it easier for him to participate in conversations. One very useful one that I liked especially was "Not make sense!"*

Pete: Yeah, that's it.

Elizabeth: I'm sleepy but I like talking with you like this. I will miss you when you leave this life and go to Mom. Will you keep talking to me then?

Pete: Yes, Sis. If I can, I will. Anyway, good night, sleep tight.

Elizabeth: You too, Bro.

S E P T E M B E R   5 ,   2 0 1 9

Putty: Hello, my dear. There are those here who would speak, perhaps your brother Pete.

Pete: Hello, Sis. I am here. I am glad to talk with you.

Elizabeth: May I ask you a question?

Pete: Yes, Sis, you and your questions. Go ahead.

Elizabeth: Are you still friends with the puppets?

Pete: Yeah, Sis. Sometimes they are around.

Elizabeth: Can you tell me more about the puppets?

Pete: What do you want to know?

Elizabeth: Do they talk with you or are they quiet?

Pete: They don't talk the way you and I talk with our speaking voices. When they talk with each other, their talk sounds like music, bells, or a bubbly creek. But they can talk with me in the way you and I are talking now—sort of mind to mind without speaking.

Elizabeth: What do they say?

Pete: Sometimes they sing little songs, not always to me but with each other.

Elizabeth: Are they like fairies?

Pete: I don't know, Sis. They are small and kind and some go with me. I like them. They sort of watch out for me.

Elizabeth: That must feel nice. Bro, how are you feeling? You bumped your teeth out somehow.

Pete: Oh, Sis. I don't really want to talk about that.

Elizabeth: Well, I think you have an appointment with the dentist to see how he can help fix your teeth. Do you want to get your teeth fixed?

Pete: I guess so, Sis. It's harder to talk, to eat as they are. I want to see Mom.

Elizabeth: Can you go see her whenever you want to?

Pete: Sometimes, yes. It is better than some days and nights now. I think you are tired. So am I, but I am life-tired. I don't want to live much longer.

Elizabeth: Why, Bro?

Pete: Because it is hard, and I like where Mom is. I want to go there.

Elizabeth: Well, I don't know for sure, but I think where Mom is is what some call heaven, and I think it's pretty nice, but I don't know for sure. I just believe that. I think I need to sleep.

Pete: Okay, Sis, sweet dreams. Bed bug bite.

S E P T E M B E R   7 ,   2 0 1 9

Putty: Hello, my dear poet. I open the gate to what voices might come in.

Pete: Hello, Sis. You are spending much time about me these days. That is okay with me if it is okay with you. I'm sorry I cannot be more present when you are with me. I do the best I can, but even if I try, it isn't always in my control. I just fade out, go elsewhere, go half asleep, travel in my mind. Not my intention. It just happens, so I am glad I can explain like this.

It seemed that Pete, when asleep, had some idea about how he was when awake. But when he was awake, there seemed to be no sign that he was aware of these sleep-time conversations.

Elizabeth: Thank you, Bro. I think I understand. Is there anything else you want to tell me?

Pete: Yes, I want to say that mostly I've had a good life and I am ready to leave.

Elizabeth: That sounds good, Bro. As for leaving, can you just decide to leave this life when you want to?

Pete: I don't know. Sometimes it seems I make decisions. Sometimes decisions are made for me.

I am ready to go. My life is difficult now and difficult for others.

Elizabeth: Is there something I can do to help make your life easier?

Pete: No, not really. These conversations are nice, and it's good to be with you. I am glad you have been my sister.

Elizabeth: I open my heart and ready my hand to write the words of anyone who would speak.

Mom: Hello, dear. Thanks for your care of your brother.

Elizabeth: Do you know what happened with Pete at night when he hurt his head, his teeth?

Mom: Oh, my dear, let me say this. Yes, Pete is vulnerable. He could tell you, of course, what happened that night. He won't. Don't press him. The primary concern is Pete's well-being.

> *As a result of this incident, a monitoring device was installed in Pete's bed so that if he got out of bed in the night, a buzzer would go off on the night staff person's desk.*

This is the middle of your night. Go back to sleep. With my love, dear, and the love of all of us who will be welcoming Pete very soon and you still many years from now.

CHAPTER THREE

BIGGER PETE SPEAKS

Elizabeth: I open my heart. My hand travels off without my conscious control. Pete or anyone?

Pete: Hello, Sis, this is Pete, or bigger than Pete, talking. Pete would want to say goodbye to you. He wants to leave his life now and wants to go wherever his self takes him next. He says he is ready. There is not much more that he wants to stay alive for. It is only the act of leaving—how to do it, how will it go, that he worries about. Maybe you can reassure him.

Here was this voice again who called himself Pete but talked about Pete as if he were someone else.

Elizabeth: I don't want to say anything to rush him ahead of his time or because I hope that he might then teach me about it or because I might be in a hurry to see his grander life after death.

Pete: Elizabeth—Sis, as he calls you—this is Pete's bigger self asking this of you. It is more than permission. It's a request.

I was beginning to hear more from and understand a bit better about this other voice identifying himself as Pete's bigger or higher self in the world of spirit.

Elizabeth: Well, then I am confused, not sure what to say or how to address any words I would say.

Pete: Just tell him/me that it is okay to leave, a good idea to leave, that you will miss him/me but that you look forward in love to talking with him in his/my afterlife.

It seemed that Bigger Pete's combining the pronouns here, such as "him/me" and "his/my" and "he/I," was an attempt to indicate something of the close relationship between Pete and Bigger Pete.

Elizabeth: Well, that is a lofty purpose so I will try.

Pete, dear Bro, if you are listening, I offer my permission for you to leave this life when you are ready to move in your spirit to your afterlife, where I believe you will see Mom and Dad and others you love, where you can be your most wonderful self, and where I hope you and I can continue to talk like this. If you do not like to think about that big change—what people call dying—that is understandable.

We don't know what it will feel like, how we will manage it, but I believe you will do beautifully, probably very sweetly and peacefully—just close your eyes and drift away from this life, leave your body, and then find the most special and beautiful self of you in a new, wonderful place. People here, like me, will cry to see you go but be glad you went when you yourself decided to go and happy believing your self will be in a beautiful new place where Mom, Dad, and others will welcome you and be so glad to see you.

What do you think about that?

Pete: Oh, Sis, thank you. It feels like you are holding my hand and hugging me and then like maybe you are not the one hugging but others. Could that be?

Elizabeth: I don't know for sure, Bro, but it sounds beautiful. You can do it. I believe you can do it beautifully and I wish you well. I believe you will be glad, very glad. So, I leave all those thoughts with you, in the peace, wisdom, and protection of what knows better than you and I how all of this works. I think that who knows better is called Love.

Elizabeth: Here I am, early morning, my hand ready to write, to hear from anyone in spirit or somewhere between here and there, like brother Pete. I surrender my hand.

Elizabeth: Pete, Bigger Pete, are you talkable?

Pete: Hi, Sis, I am here—this is Pete, Bigger Pete, your brother and then some, traveling between here and there. I am learning so many things—who I am, who I really and truly am. I had forgotten so much in my restricted life. I am a being that exists far beyond what most people know of me. I am happy to learn of who I truly am, of who I can be, all that I can do. If in my life as Pete, I could do these things, be this bigger self I had forgotten, had only, at best, the occasional glimpse. The difference, the gap, between Pete and Bigger Pete is huge. Bigger Pete is so much more than just Pete, but I'll call myself, for the time being, Bigger Pete, because you know me as Pete, I know me as Pete, this life I've been living, but it's such a small part. And here is the thing, Sis, and maybe I should call you Bigger Sis. I believe everyone—I know everyone—is the same way. Any one life on Earth is just a small part—an important part but just still a small part of all that one truly is. Sis, Bigger Sis, I have to tell you—this truly is grand.

It is a miracle, you could even say, to see the beautiful, wonderful of . . . what can I call it? You are the writer. You must write this down. You must tell other people. People must know, they must be aware of the much bigger story. And you, the writer, can tell it.

Elizabeth: Well, Pete, Bigger Pete, if you tell me, I will write it and see about publishing it.

Pete: Good, that is good. Now I have to see how I can tell it. It is so much more than I had dreamed of, so much more than I could have guessed. If I knew this before, if some part of me knew it, I had forgotten. But I'll say this. This life, this life after life, is, well, amazing. Why people decide to be born into life on Earth I'm still figuring out. If you will listen and write it, I promise to tell you all that I am learning.

Elizabeth: Pete, Bigger Pete, Bro, this is exciting, and I promise to you that I'll do my best.

Pete: I want to be here in this bigger life all the time, but I will feel better about my coming here if you will tell others what I can tell you.

Elizabeth: That's a deal.

Pete: I think this is all that I can do now.

Elizabeth: Okay, then goodbye. Until next time, but what do I call you if you're bigger now than just Pete?

Pete: How about Bigger Pete, just for now?

Elizabeth: Okay, Bigger Pete. Until next time.

S E P T E M B E R   1 8 ,   2 0 1 9

Elizabeth: I am here, to write. I surrender myself to the great unknown I wish to know better.

Pete: Hi, Sis—this is Pete Bigger Pete, flying about, traveling to strange and wonderful places. I cannot tell you all the things I see and hear, but I wish I could. You would be amazed. It's always good to see Mom when I can.

Elizabeth: Can you just wish to see her and then you can see her?

Pete: Not always, but sometimes it seems like that. And Dad, too. But there are others I haven't seen before. And they are not really people like Mom and Dad but more like big colors or light or energy, but they feel like people, like someone or something that loves you and speaks but not usual speaking—more like they think and then I somehow know what they think.

I came to realize that Pete may have been visiting his afterlife while he was still living. It didn't seem as if he was thinking of it as his afterlife but just a place he was visiting and then could describe.

It feels like they hug me or carry me, take me places or allow me to see things I have not seen before, or maybe that I haven't seen for a very long time. It makes me feel good, but it is strange. Like a dream, feels like home I have forgotten. Not like where I live when awake.

Not like where I was born with you all, but another home, hard to say.

Elizabeth: And what are you like when you're there?

Pete: Oh, I am just fine. I can see and hear and feel and move so easily. I am me, myself, but a wonderful self. Yes, I am Pete, but not just Pete. Pete is just a part, a small part. I am bigger, stronger, peaceful, and happy. It feels like I can go anywhere, do anything, or be happy just as I am. It is wonderful, no aches or pains. No difficulties. I don't need to do anything, just be and be and be who I am, just as I am, and it's fine. Does that make sense?

Elizabeth: It sounds wonderful. I'd like to see it.

Pete: Well, Sis, I think you can. I think you already know about this, but you see when I wake up, then I am Pete again—little old Pete in my bed. That's familiar but it has its ups and downs, and sometimes it's hard to be just my old familiar self.

So, Sis, I would say it is better for you to be where you are. I think it's better for each of us to do what is best for each of us. You don't have to be like me. I don't have to be like you. It is more amazing for us all to be our little selves that are also just a little piece of something much bigger and beautiful. I love you, Sis. You know something, Sis? When I am in this wonderful place or space, everything is love. Everything. That's what makes it feel so good. It is just all around. It's all love. Oh, Sis. Can I just be here?

Elizabeth: Bro, I am happy you are so happy and somewhere so amazing.

Pete: Sis, I think this is all that I can say now. Thank you, Sis. Thank you, Sis. Thank you, Sis.

Unidentified spirits: Elizabeth, dear Elizabeth, you too are traveling while you sit in your chair. You too get to see and hear just as your brother does, but he will be leaving there to come here. You will stay where you are. Not your time to come here. Your work is to write, to connect, to communicate. It is good work and very much needed. People want to hear, to read the words you are writing. Keep writing. This is our encouragement. Allow others to go. Let them tell you and you write it. That is all for now.

Elizabeth: Wow! Thank you, whoever you are!

Elizabeth: I surrender myself to allow my hand to write words.

Putty: Hello, sweet woman.

Pete: Hello, Sis. I am here. I always like this talking with you. It makes me feel like myself, but not just little and fading self as Pete, but a bigger self—me when I am more than just the Pete near the end of Pete's life. That life is finishing. But, Sis, I am not so scared now. I have an idea, a picture of my next bigger life after life as Pete. And Sis, talking with you makes me less scared.

Elizabeth: I am glad to hear you are not scared.

Pete: Sis, my life as Pete wasn't so bad. I may have been much for others to care for, but I hope that I have not hurt others. I am glad for the family I was born in. Mom was amazing. Always she wanted the best for me, even when she was tough and insistent. We had our battles, but I know she wanted the best for me. She was relentless on that. Of course, it would make her look better if I looked and acted better, but her best self wanted the best for me. So, I thank her and when I go to live with her, I can thank her still more.

Dad did what he could. He was different. He tried, but I guess as a man, as a father, he and I had a different relationship. When I was little, he always wanted to call me Pete Repeat. I didn't like that. I made that clear, but he latched onto that name. I think he thought it was clever or cute. I didn't. Oh well. Sometimes he didn't know how best to be a father to me, but he always meant well. I think his squabbles, his parting ways with Mom, complicated the thing. I hope all that is past, that maybe we all learned something. It's about learning, isn't it, Sis? You are the teacher. You are not teaching in schools anymore, but you are still teaching.

It was now well over ten years since I had retired early from college teaching to help Pete in the inevitable Alzheimer's decline.

When you write down our conversations like this and let others read them, it'll be like teaching too. We are teaching together, you and I. Hey, that's amazing, Sis! I can be a teacher too.

Elizabeth: Bro, you are an amazing teacher. I have learned so much from you.

Pete: Thanks, Sis. You haven't always had an easy time with me. I know that I can be stubborn. But that's how I get to have some force. I do not have so many ways to be strong. Sometimes saying no can be very strong or at least help me to feel strong when, otherwise, I don't feel strong, or people don't think I am strong. Does that make sense?

Elizabeth: I guess so. I'm thinking about it. I am glad you can tell me this.

Pete: That's why I like talking like this. I can say things like this that I cannot say as just Pete, but I can say them as Bigger Pete. Let's talk again.

Elizabeth: Okay, Bro.

S E P T E M B E R 2 3 , 2 0 1 9

Elizabeth: I am open to anything. My heart is open, my hand is ready to write.

Pete: Hi, Sis. Thank you for this talk. Do you have one of your questions for me?

Elizabeth: Yes, Bro. I want to ask you again about your puppets. Can you tell me more about them?

Pete: Oh, Sis, the puppets are my friends. I can't remember when they first came, but I think it was when I started having real trouble. My thinking was hard, a problem. I could tell my thinking wasn't as good because my talking wasn't as good either. It became hard to say what I wanted to say. It's even harder now. Much easier to say nothing at all. I couldn't do anything about that. It just started happening. It was easier to be quiet or to show signs than to talk. That's why this talking with you is so good. No problem at all. I can talk with you without really talking.

The puppets don't really talk, either. They make noises but their language is different, pretty, like music, but I can sometimes understand because I can understand their thinking. Some people now seem to understand my thinking even when I don't talk. You know, Sis, what helps that? Love and caring. When people are loving and caring, they can understand other people even when there is no talking. That's what the puppets do. They are loving and caring. I don't always understand them, especially when they talk with each other, but they can understand me and my thoughts. And they are good friends because they keep me company. And that helps a lot.

Elizabeth: What do you mean—helps in what way?

Pete: It helps to feel less lonely. Talk connects people. People rely on talk. With no talk, it's lonely but it doesn't have to be quite as lonely. Loving and caring has other ways too than just talking. Do you understand, Sis?

Elizabeth: Yes, Bro. You tell it beautifully, and I think I am learning another something from you. So, the puppets help you feel less lonely?

Pete: Oh, yes, Sis. They are amazing. You want to know what they look like? Mostly, they are small, not tall at all, but they can make themselves look bigger if they need to.

Elizabeth: Why would they need to?

Pete: When they want me to notice or pay attention more, or they have something important to show me or tell me, but they don't like to do that. I think it's like their way of shouting, and shouting isn't nice, shouldn't be necessary, but sometimes, just a few times, it is. Names? Well, sort of. But I don't usually have to call them. They seem to come when it is helpful for me for them to come. Sometimes I think they make up names just to make it easier for me, like that time they were keeping me awake and I couldn't sleep, remember, Sis?

Pete was talking about that time when he visited us, and I went to check on him late because I had heard noise from his room.

Elizabeth: When one of them, Mary, was in your bed and keeping you awake?

Pete: Yeah, Sis. You came and stayed next to me so there wouldn't be room for her until I fell asleep. That worked. She left me so I could sleep, but I think some of them like being around me the way I like being around them.

Elizabeth: That sounds nice, Bro.

Pete: Well, they are my friends. They are different but I like them, and they keep me company.

And sometimes it's nice not to feel so alone, so all by myself all the time.

Elizabeth: Are they still around?

Pete: Oh, yeah, Sis. Except not so much right now when I'm talking with you, but I think our talking right now is done, isn't it, Sis?

Elizabeth: It can be, Bro. But I am happy to talk again with you whenever you want to.

Pete: Thanks, Sis. You are a good sister. Goodbye for now.

Elizabeth: Take good care of your wonderful self, Bro.

SEPTEMBER 25, 2019

Elizabeth: I am here with open heart and ready hand to write what words will come.

Pete: Hi, Sis. Pete is sleeping, but this is Bigger Pete, who can speak. It is good to talk like this. And I will be able to talk with you like this even when Pete leaves life for the afterlife, although it may be different or take some time to make that connection.

Elizabeth: I trust what you are saying, but how do you know this? I don't understand Pete and Bigger Pete very well, I guess. Can you help me to understand?

Pete: Sure, Sis, and I'll call you that because that is what Pete calls you. I, Bigger Pete, a good name, I guess, is the Pete you know, but more than the Pete you know. I know things that Pete doesn't know or doesn't remember as Pete. Pete knows his own life as Pete and is now in the process of traveling, you might say, and learning and remembering that he is and has been and will be more than just his life as Pete. He is curious as he learns, but right now, I am speaking to you as his self that is aware of more than he is usually aware. I can talk with you as Pete, the Pete you know, or as Bigger Pete, which is going to be who he grows back into being when he leaves his life as just Pete. Do you understand?

Elizabeth: I think so. And I guess that is what happens for all of us after physical life, yes?

Pete: Yes, that's pretty much right, but each situation has its own qualities. When people lose their faculties, often at the end of life or earlier or throughout any particular life, the gap may be larger between their physical life and their bigger life, as we are calling it.

Elizabeth: You sound so wise.

Pete: Not like the Pete you know, right? It's okay. I understand. But that is exactly the idea. There is, in Pete's situation, quite a big difference between Pete who has limited abilities, especially now, and me, Bigger Pete, who is hardly familiar at all to you. And that is why I think it is taking some time for Pete himself now to make sense of himself as Pete and me as Bigger Pete. Imagine it! But he is doing splendidly. I am doing splendidly. I should say, we're all doing splendidly.

Life on Earth is not easy, but most do their best, and after life on Earth or when people get a glimpse of life beyond, it is rather a lot to understand. I hope this helps to explain. Because just as I don't sound like the brother Pete you know, just think how I must sound to Pete himself.

Quite a puzzle, yes? Anyway, that is what is happening. Now I'll stop talking. We can talk again.

Elizabeth: Wow, thanks, Pete Bigger Pete. Amazing! Until next time then!

SEPTEMBER 26, 2019

Putty: Good morning, my dear young poet-author-wonder woman.

Elizabeth: Now you're teasing me!

Putty: Only a little. You are wonderful in your dedication.

Elizabeth: Well, thanks.

Putty: Shall I open the gate?

Elizabeth: Please, and thank you, Putty. I'd like to hug you—you, the wonder man.

Pete: Hi, Sis, I was hoping you'd call for me. I am here but just for a little bit. I feel topsy-turvy.

Elizabeth: In a good way, Bro, or not?

Pete: Sis, I am confused, not quite sure where I am or who I am.

Elizabeth: Well, Bro, you are my wonderful brother Pete. And I think you are Pete in a much bigger way too that maybe you are now remembering. Maybe that is a little confusing. Is that it?

Pete: Yeah, sort of like that. Sis, I feel like, well, don't know how to say it, but when I wake up in my bed, I feel small, confused, not able to think right or talk right like I used to.

Elizabeth: Oh, Bro, I give you a big hug. That must be frustrating.

Pete: Yeah, Sis. I just want to go back to sleep. Then maybe those feelings go away and something nicer happens.

Elizabeth: Bro, do you want me to say what I think is happening?

Pete: Sure, Sis, go ahead.

Elizabeth: I think when you go to sleep, your body stays quiet on your bed, but your mind, your thinking, gets to travel in spirit, and you also get to be a bigger you, Bigger Pete—that is Pete, but just bigger, stronger, and you aren't so confused. Does that make sense?

Pete: I think so, Sis.

Elizabeth: Well, Bro, when you do feel confused or don't feel so good, just imagine I am holding your hand, that I am with you. My body is not with you, but my love is with you. Does that make sense?

Pete: Yeah, Sis. Sounds nice.

Elizabeth: And Bro, wherever you are, awake or asleep, Pete or Bigger Pete, I think a lot of people are loving you like Mom, Dad, many people who are no longer living, and many people who are living. Love is all around you. You are not alone.

Pete: Oh, Sis, I don't know. I feel kind of lost, alone on a big, lonely road and I don't know where it is going, where I am going.

Elizabeth: That must be hard, but remember, Bro, even though you can't see us, there are many who are with you, loving you, supporting you on that road where you are. And you will not feel lonely for long. It will pass, and all will be well, beautiful, and wonderful. Can you keep that in your thinking?

Pete: Oh, thank you, Sis. Thank you, Sis. I feel better already . . . I think.

Elizabeth: Good, I'm glad. You are not alone but, in a place, always with love all around. Until next time we talk, sweet dreams.

Pete: Thanks, Sis.

S E P T E M B E R   2 7 ,   2 0 1 9

Elizabeth: Good morning. My hand is ready to write. I am eager to hear from anyone—Pete?

Pete: Sis, it's me—happy to talk with you. I feel better today. Don't worry about me. It's just sometimes I feel lost and alone, as if in darkness. You help me feel better. I think I am ready for whatever comes next for me. I don't really have much in my life that makes me want to live it each day, but I don't want to die. I am a little scared of dying—not much right now, but a little.

Elizabeth: Yes, Bro, I think most of us think death is scary, but I am learning that what waits for us all after death is a wonderful afterlife. That's what I believe. I think that when you have had enough of this life and are ready to go on, you will, but I don't know how that decision is made.

If you know or learn it later, I hope you will tell me.

Pete: If I can, I will, Sis.

O C T O B E R   1 ,   2 0 1 9

Elizabeth: I call for those who wish to speak. Pete, are you there and wanting to talk with me?

Putty: Hello, my dear poet woman. We are all around you, support you in more ways than you can imagine. Now let's see if your brother wishes to speak first before those fully in spirit.

Pete: Hi, Sis. I am here.

Elizabeth: Hello, Bro. Are you sleeping? Or where are you?

Pete: Sis, my body, my old body is on my bed. My thinking can go off like dreams anywhere. I can talk with you.

Elizabeth: Maybe soon you will wake up and have a fine day.

Pete: No, Sis, I don't want to wake up. I don't know what the day will be, but I know where I am now is nicer, easier. So, I would like to sleep longer.

Elizabeth: Where are you, Bro?

Pete: Hard to say, Sis. In a way, nowhere and everywhere. If I think of you, I can be in your house in my chair in the kitchen or anywhere. I like my bed in your house.

Elizabeth: I'm glad, Bro. Can you go now in your thinking wherever you want to be?

Pete: Sort of, but not exactly. I can't make myself go places, but sometimes it seems I can think myself there, but not at all when I'm awake. It's a little like floating, but it's like someone or something else is also deciding where I will go.

Elizabeth: Oh. Who is the someone else?

Pete: I'm not sure, Sis. It's sort of me, sort of not me. Bigger, stronger, but gentle.

Elizabeth: Bro, do you like how you yourself are when you are sleeping?

Pete: Sis, I forget that my body is sleeping. I am just me, until you start asking all your questions and we talk like this. I like talking like this, but I can't always answer all your questions. Sis?

Elizabeth: Yes?

Pete: I want to tell you something.

Elizabeth: Okay.

Pete: I think my body is going to stop soon. It is tired.

Elizabeth: Can you feel that? How do you know that?

Pete: I don't know how I know it. Something else knows it—sort of something in my body and sort of not in my body. Like my body is tired even after I sleep and just wants to stop. But there's still something else that doesn't want to stop.

Elizabeth: Bro, I am just guessing but I think the part that doesn't want to stop may be what people call the soul. And I think the soul can keep going and is very happy to keep going when the body stops. Before, you called that Bigger Pete, if you remember that, yes?

Pete: Oh, Sis, there are so many things I don't know or don't know well. Sometimes I feel I am smarter and know more stuff. Other times I don't know or it's too hard to even try to know.

Elizabeth: Well, Bro, I'm not sure I understand exactly, but I think the way you tell it is very good.

Pete: Thanks, Sis. Can we talk again?

Elizabeth: Of course, Bro, of course. Let's talk again. We'll say bye for now.

O C T O B E R   1 ,   2 0 1 9

Elizabeth: I am here, ready to write.

Pete: Hi, Sis. Want to talk?

Elizabeth: Sure, Bro, what would you like to say?

Pete: Sis, I wonder about things that I cannot talk about.

Elizabeth: Can you talk about them the way we talk like this? Is it hard to describe what you want to say, or are you worried about what I or someone else might say?

Pete: Well, Sis, I don't know, but there are many things I think about but cannot say about them. I don't know how to say what I am thinking.

Elizabeth: Bro, that's true for many people. Sometimes it just seems impossible to say things we are thinking. But if you want to try just a little, just here, just you and me, I will listen and try to understand.

Pete: Okay, Sis. I would like to say how it feels when I am sort of in the world and then I am sort of in another world where sometimes I see Mom. I want to tell you, but I can't really. It's so amazing and I don't know the words for it.

Elizabeth: Bro, I'm sorry.

I felt frustrated too by Pete's inability to describe better how he felt between worlds, but it seemed anyone would have the same difficulty in trying to describe the different worlds in ordinary language.

OCTOBER 2, 2019

Elizabeth: Hello, spirits. I am here, hand ready to write.

Mom: Hello, dear.

Elizabeth: Yesterday they called to say that Pete tried to open the van door from inside while the van was moving. It could be confusion, but I wonder what Pete was thinking.

Mom: Well, you may think when we die, we become amazingly omniscient, but that's <u>not</u> the case. I, for one, couldn't say what he was thinking.

Unidentified spirits: We come as a group to commend you and your work. You will find people are interested. Oh, and pay attention to politics and such but don't allow yourself to become too distracted or despairing. Others will tend to that.

Elizabeth: Thank you. Is that it or is there more?

Unidentified spirits: Oh, plenty more, but for now, see if your brother wishes to speak.

Elizabeth: I am ready to write more, especially if Pete or Bigger Pete wishes to speak.

Pete: Hi, Sis, it's me. Thank you for talking with me. Not many people do now because I do not say much. I am slow and getting slower. Usually, people do not want to wait.

Elizabeth: Oh, Bro, I think I am one of those people. I get impatient, want things to move faster. If you and I sit together and talk, I know now it takes longer for you to listen, think, and then say something. So, I am sorry when I get impatient because sometimes you <u>do</u> have something to say. So, this kind of talking between us is easier, isn't it?

Pete: Yeah, Sis. I don't have any trouble talking this way. The way you talk and the way I talk are not so very different when we do this.

Now it seemed almost as if there were three versions of Pete. There was Pete when he was awake but, due to Alzheimer's, had become unable to converse. There was Pete when he was asleep, the familiar Pete, but somehow able to converse. Then Bigger Pete appeared, who described himself as Pete's higher self—Pete but who sounded different—wiser, more formal—than the familiar Pete.

Elizabeth: I have a question, Bro. May I ask?

Pete: So many questions! I call you Question Sis, ha ha! Go ahead, Sis— what is your question at this time?

Elizabeth: Bro, do you remember calling yourself Bigger Pete when you were Pete as I know you but also a lot more—bigger, stronger, and knowing very many things?

Pete: I don't know, Sis. It sounds okay, but, well, that is one of your questions I cannot answer very well. At least not right now. Anything else?

Elizabeth: Not right now. How about instead of a question, I just send you a hug?

Pete: Yeah, Sis. That's good. I like hugs, lots of hugs, long hugs, hugs are good. Thanks, Sis.

OCTOBER 4, 2019

Elizabeth: Good morning, spirits. I am ready to write. I surrender my arm.

Pete: And I am here, too—the one you are calling Bigger Pete, your brother Pete included. I know you want so much to know how this all works—Pete, Bigger Pete, the world you know as the world of spirit. I can tell you this. No spirit has a plan to keep things secret from you, but we do know that it is hard to understand while in a physical life on Earth how the world of spirit functions or just is. But as you ask, and we know you are so curious, we do our best to explain what you already know in your bigger self, too.

Elizabeth: "We"?

Pete: You see, even that is hard to explain. I, myself, that is really more than one self. I am a total of many lives, experiences, and more than the lives lived physically on Earth. I am also including the lives between which may be long and many. So, you see, it is almost better to say "we" than "I," just as you are trying to distinguish in your own words "Bigger Pete" and "Pete."

Those words, that distinction, is a good one and shows that you grasp some of what I am explaining, what we are explaining. If you like, as you write, you may want to use "we" when Bigger Pete speaks and "I" when the Pete you know speaks. Some describe this difference as levels, hierarchies, and so forth.

Then there is something else, too. When I/we say "we," it also includes those in spirit who merge and depart from the core me/we. That is (and this may be still harder to fathom), the lines between one entity and another in spirit are more fluid, not like the hard and fast physicality you are familiar with as a body on physical Earth.

Let's see if I can explain this part. Okay, let's try this: When you make love or are really truly in love, the lines blur between yourself and the other whom you love, yes? You know this experience, yes? The line that divides you, that distinguishes you from the loved one becomes more fluid, not so hard, fast, and impenetrable. You merge together somewhat. Does that make sense?

Elizabeth: Yes.

Pete: Well, the world of spirit is Love. All of us, you might say, are swimming in love. We do not always need to insist on such divisions, separations, lines of distinction between us. It's more fluid, so when we choose words, sometimes "we" makes more sense than just "I," but of course, the main thing in language is communication, so any speaking to another must take into account what will make sense to that other. So much of any choosing of words is about choosing what will facilitate understanding. I hope this is clear. See, now I say "I," not "we" because you were questioning "we" when I used it.

Elizabeth: Wow! Okay, that's very clear, and I have to say you must indeed be what I am calling, and you have called "Bigger Pete," because I'm not sure Pete as Pete could or would have said all that way.

Pete: It's true and I know you were asking the Pete part of me to explain. The Pete part of me by himself would probably choose not to even try. That is, in part, due to the fact that his own language, especially his speaking aloud, is not easy these days because of what's going on in his physical self. But his mental and spiritual self can speak well, as you have seen when the physical apparatus of speech is not part of the matter.

Elizabeth: Wow, okay.

***

OCTOBER 6, 2019

Elizabeth: I am open to anyone's words with my heart open, hand ready.

Putty: Hello, my dear. Yes, it's good to follow these routines that allow you to connect to the world of spirit. You are more adept now and more trusting in what is ready to come to you.

Congratulations! That is the result of your years of work. Now I will open the gate, my dear.

Pete: I am Bigger Pete, a useful moniker. I am happy to speak with you anytime, as Pete is. It is not easy to explain how Pete and Bigger Pete fit together, but for now, I am speaking as Bigger Pete, a voice which, for you, comes to you not from the physical Earth but beyond. Pete, as you know him, as your brother, lives a physical life on Earth as you do. But he is part of something bigger that we are calling Bigger Pete. Bigger Pete includes Pete but also includes other lives, lives between lives, and more. So, I am speaking as Bigger Pete, but I am focusing on Pete, so what I have to say is about Pete, not about other lives than Pete. Understand?

Elizabeth: I think so. I hope so.

What I was understanding was that this Bigger Pete included but was not limited to the Pete whom I knew as my brother. However, this Bigger Pete seemed to have none of the Down syndrome or Alzheimer's limitations of my brother. Rather he was knowledgeable and well-spoken and apparently had had other lives as well as the one as my brother Pete.

Pete: Pete has been moving closer to the end of his life as Pete (as you all are, of course) on Earth, but he has moved closer, then farther, then closer again, not necessarily in total but certainly in both body and spirit. His physical body gets stronger, gets weaker, gets stronger in a cycle that is slowing, approaching physical death. Mentally, he has been afraid of the end of his life, quite understandably, but on another plane, he has been exploring (while his physical body sleeps) what his afterlife will be.

As I have said, the difference between Pete's life, especially now with its limitations, and Bigger Pete is a big difference and not easy for him to navigate. But he is doing this—navigating between life and afterlife, between Pete and his bigger soul-spirit self that you are calling Bigger Pete. His adjustment, therefore, to his afterlife is likely to be much bigger than others. But he is already engaged in doing this adjustment while he is still living as Pete. And I can tell you that he is assisted in this effort by many here in spirit, and he is assisted by those in his life on Earth.

So, he is very definitely in an in-between state, a transitional state. At any time, he could cross over as his adjustment will involve further adjustment. When that time comes, which I cannot tell, could be any time. Does this make sense to you?

Elizabeth: Yes, I think so, and I am glad to learn more how this all happens.

Pete: Your part in this has been magnificent. Not only are you keeping watch, watching his care, but also your being able to have these conversations as part of his transition, his adjustment process. And while it's only dim, he has a slim awareness of his other bigger self. And, as he has said, he gives full consent for this writing to become public. It will serve many and I, as well as others, are grateful. We thank you and do all we can to support you in this effort. So that is all I will say now. Go in peace and love.

O C T O B E R   8 ,   2 0 1 9

Elizabeth: I am ready to write. Hand is ready, heart is open.

Pete: Thank you, Sis, for our talking. I am fine. I am fine. I am just going along, doing the days, doing the nights.

Elizabeth: How do you feel, Bro?

Pete: I feel good, I guess. Tired but okay. It is hard to get comfortable sometimes. I don't need much. I am okay. You are good, Sis. I know you care and do things for me even when I do not see you here. It's good we can talk like this. I am resting. I like to sleep. It feels better than being awake.

By now, with his advanced dementia, Pete was sleeping more hours during the day. It was obvious that negotiating his daily life when awake was becoming even more exhausting.

Awake is okay, but it's so hard now. I need so much help. What would I do if I had to do everything myself? I don't know. This is what getting old is, right, Sis?

Elizabeth: Bro, I guess some of it. People have different ways of getting old in their bodies because bodies aren't all the same.

Pete: Sis, are you getting old?

Elizabeth: Oh, yes, I'm getting old. I can't see as well. I get tired more easily. Stuff like that.

And, oh, I have trouble remembering things. How about you?

Pete: Sis, I can remember some things but not everything. I almost remember many things but then can't actually remember the whole thing, just bits or nothing. Some days it bothers me. And it takes so long to remember. Takes so long to do everything.

Elizabeth: Bro, if there isn't anything more, I am going to go to sleep.

Pete: Sis, have a good sleep. I am having a good sleep. Bed bug bite.

OCTOBER 9, 2019

Elizabeth: Good morning, spirits, or any who are around somehow.

Putty: Oh, we are around. This is Putty, of course, but there's a crowd.

Elizabeth: Really? Who then speaks first?

Putty: Leave that to me, dear, and them.

Elizabeth: Yes, okay. Thank you.

Mom: Hello, dear. Now about Pete—yes, he's coasting. He has small daily ups and downs and can continue like this for a while. You have seen how years (your years) ago, I said he was at the end of his life, coming to us soon. But he has had quite a few ups and downs, close calls, and rallies. It is not a steady decline with death at the end, nor are accidental deaths as neat as they seem. Even when the medical signs say that death has occurred, what happens for any one person can involve a more drawn-out process. One shouldn't focus so absolutely on one point of death.

Pete has been visiting what will be his afterlife, trying to work out what it means. He cannot tell you this. He can hardly get it all himself, and he doesn't have the thinking or words to tell you now, but he can tell you much by this communication, these conversations you're having. And my dear, these conversations are helping him with the transition as much as you benefit too from what you are learning. He has guides here. You are a guide there, and all of it helps him. That is why I and others keep commending you and your efforts. Not many would rise so early just to sit and do this writing which, no doubt, would strike many as bizarre. But you do it and it's good. So enough of me. I'll be quiet now, let others speak.

Pete: Hello, Elizabeth. This is Pete's larger self—Bigger Pete, as we've been saying. The Pete part of me is ready to move on. If he could, he would thank many who have made his life easier, including you. He may be able still to do that, but I suspect he'll want to do that, find ways to do that, when he leaves that life, merges with me—his bigger self. That's all I'll say now but do call on me again. I am happy to help this project of yours. Love and peace to you.

Elizabeth: Thank you, Bigger Pete.

As Pete declined and I needed to pay more attention to his care, I was also taking time to do this writing—"this project," as Bigger Pete called it—and my poetry writing ended. Earlier in the year, a new book of my tanka poetry had been published, which seemed likely to be my last poetry book, at least for the foreseeable future.

*After retiring from teaching anthropology at the college and taking
up poetry, I had had a number of requests to teach poetry classes,
some of which I accepted, but those too fell by the wayside, as Pete's
care and this writing took precedence.*

OCTOBER 12, 2019

Elizabeth: Here I am, ready to write the words of anyone who wishes to
speak.

Pete: Hi, Sis, it's Pete, well, the one you call Bigger Pete, including Pete,
the Pete you know best.

Elizabeth: I do not fully understand what Pete knows of Bigger Pete and
vice versa. Can you explain?

Pete: I have explained some. It is no different in its essence from others.
What makes this relationship different is that Pete has physical limitations that mean he cannot, in his physical body, fully understand
Bigger Pete. Most people on Earth cannot either, but with Pete, the
gap is bigger because he has the cognitive limitations he has had since
birth and now this dementia. So in a way, I, as Bigger Pete, know
more about Pete than Pete knows about Bigger Pete. But there are
also some things he knows that I, as Bigger Pete, do not.

Elizabeth: Such as?

Pete: He knows what it <u>feels</u> like to be in the body of Pete, its pains and
pleasures. He knows what it feels like in the body to care for others
and that others care for him, like you, his sister.

I, as Bigger Pete, know some of that, but he knows that better.
He also—Pete, that is—has fears that I do not have, such as the fear
of death. When his physical body sleeps, his mental, his spiritual
aspects, are aware of more, and he can do things like mental travel
that he cannot do when awake and limited in the physical world.
And physically, he is very limited.

His body is not doing well. It will not serve him much longer,
and when it no longer works to keep him alive, he will break into

a fuller knowing as me, Bigger Pete, who will not be limited by the limits of his Earthly physical form. It is true that now he could completely decide that there is nothing other than Pete. That is, no Bigger Pete, as many other people do. But when asleep, he has been traveling, learning, making the transition to his larger self, so if he could say so when awake, he would probably not deny completely the possibility of Bigger Pete, but he just couldn't talk coherently about all this.

You can see the gap I am speaking of because you hear me now, as Bigger Pete, which sounds nothing like Pete, the brother you know. So, you have your own struggle putting Pete and Bigger Pete together in any meaningful way. It's why you keep asking about it, but you do not have the particular cognitive limitations Pete has.

In fact, physically and mentally, you are in a good situation to understand all this better than Pete and even better than many people. Also, because of your life experience and now your willingness to write this down, you have the unique capability of coming to understand it well enough to help others understand and also to help you understand the big effort that is involved in the transition Pete is undergoing. Whew! That is probably much more than you wanted as an answer.

Elizabeth: Not at all. I am glad for it. Thank you. It does seem there is an intermediary or in-between state of Pete. It seems in these writings that there is Pete awake with his physical limitations but also Pete who, when asleep, can talk with me through this writing but is yet not you as Bigger Pete.

Pete: Ah, yes, very perceptive. That is correct. He is more mentally capable in his, what we might call, dream state.

OCTOBER 19, 2019

Elizabeth: I am here, ready to write. My arm goes on its own.

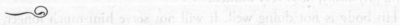

Pete: Hi, Sis, as he calls you. This is Bigger Pete, as he calls me, his bigger self. I am so glad you are doing this writing. It will be important for many, more than you think. Do you have questions?

Elizabeth: Yes, of course, always many. May I ask?

Pete: Please do.

Elizabeth: If you, Bigger Pete, are more than just Pete, are you also other lives that Pete has lived?

Pete: Oh yes. I have lived many, but what can I say? Why do you ask?

Elizabeth: I ask because I found so much help in discovering my own past lives. I guess I am curious what might, from other lives, help to understand this one of his.

Pete: Ah, then, good reason. Because if one is able to know one's other lives, it can be difficult, wrenching even sometimes, to learn of those things. Yes, there have been many, and this is hard to explain well in this writing with you.

Elizabeth: Why?

Pete: Several reasons. You learned of your lives with someone who guided you, someone who eased you through the rough parts.

Some of those past lives are chronicled in the book Journeys with Fortune: A Tale of Other Lives, *where a professional hypnotist served as one guide and Fortune served as a guide in the realm of spirit.*

I am not such a guide. Oh, I could tell details—what, when, and where—but I couldn't soften hard edges for you. And there have been hard edges. As rough as this life has been, it pales beside some of the others. It would pain you to know details. I must tell you, this life as Pete has not been easy. But what is important is that with all the limitations, lifelong and now, there has always been help. And that is the key. We all can endure more if we help each other. This is a big lesson, and some want so much independence they cannot accept help. The life as Pete could be a lesson to others on this if people, if others, thought about that. That's what I'll say to your question for now.

Elizabeth: Well, thank you. Amazing again.

OCTOBER 20, 2019

Elizabeth: Here I am, ready for guidance about Pete.

Mom: Hello, dear. Thank you for looking out for Pete, for handling things so beautifully. It isn't always as easy as you make it seem.

Elizabeth: I'm jangled.

Mom: Yes, dear, understandable. But dear, you know you should know Pete is getting ready to leave. It has been back and forth over all this time. At some point, it will happen. You'll get the call. You will do your best. I know you will. You have the strength, and you will manage. I'll be rooting for you from here. And I'll be welcoming Pete. He will be well welcomed. That I can guarantee. You will probably hear from him.

Elizabeth: I have been.

Mom: I mean after his physical life is over.

Elizabeth: Oh.

Mom: I know you have had—are having—conversations together but not tonight. His attention is elsewhere now. But call on him tomorrow. He will be glad and can talk to you then.

Elizabeth: Okay. How do you know all this?

Mom: Well, I can't really explain, but dear, after all, I gave birth to him. His welfare is my concern. I don't need to tell you that.

Elizabeth: No, but I guess I needed a nudge.

Mom: That's okay. That's all.

OCTOBER 22, 2019

Elizabeth: I surrender myself and allow my arm to write.

Putty: Hello, my dear. I am here, your gatekeeper, happy to guard at the gate.

Elizabeth: You are doing a wonderful job all these years. No problems, thanks to you, but a far cry, I think, from who you were in life and maybe are or wish to be now. I thank you.

Putty: Oh, well said, my dear. Rest assured, I do this entirely of my own volition and am as curious as you are about who shows up to speak. So, I open the gate, yes?

Elizabeth: Yes, thank you, Putty.

Pete: Hi, Sis, it's Pete—Bigger Pete, you might say. Pete is asleep. He could speak now this way to you. Maybe he will, but I am here and wish to speak.

Elizabeth: Hello, Bigger Pete.

Pete: Do you have questions? You often do.

Elizabeth: Yes, what happened on Sunday to Pete? He went to the hospital for hours because of his red, swollen foot.

Pete: Yes, his foot was swollen. And yes, they did no tests, didn't keep him. The medical people cannot treat what is metaphysical. Pete's body is slowly saying goodbye. Pete, in his thinking, which isn't so good these days, wants to stick with the life as he knows it. He has been traveling back and forth, but for some, it isn't easy to let go, to say, "Okay, I let go."

Elizabeth: This is hard to write. My eyes are watering, not crying, but watering.

Pete: Are you sure it's not crying? Maybe, for you, time for a little let go, yes?

Elizabeth: Why?

Pete: Oh, Sis, as he calls you, who is more stubborn—Pete or Sis? Hmmm. Let me say this: Why not you go crawl back in bed? You can come back to this later.

OCTOBER 22, 2019

Elizabeth: I am ready to sleep, but I'll try to stay awake. I allow my arm to go on its own.

Pete: Hi, Sis.

Elizabeth: Pete or Bigger Pete?

Pete: Well, really, we are the same. Pete is a part of me—where I am alive now on Earth, although Pete is quite asleep. He is liking the world of spirit more and more. Each time he wakes up and has to maneuver himself in his physical life, it feels difficult. Of course, he likes all the help but would rather be strong and independent. His physical body is not in balance. One part then another goes a bit off and that affects the whole body.

Elizabeth: What is most important to help him now?

Pete: Well, he does have those helping with bathing, with dressing, with eating, with moving. He can do less now.

One of the challenges for me when Pete was with me was to remind myself to slow down and allow whatever time it took help him with dressing, bathing, eating, and even my speaking with him. When I remembered to, I consciously slowed my speed of talking and tried to keep things simple. If I didn't, I would often see Pete tuning me out.

That is what is happening so the help he has on all those things is important. He cannot hold an extended conversation. He can hold hands. The body does not decline all at once, equal in every way. Vulnerable parts start to work less well—feet, brain, eyes, ears. He will accept help. He knows he needs it, can't do everything on his own. Does that answer your question?

Elizabeth: Well, yes, and then some. Thank you. I don't know what to say, but I guess you, Bigger Pete, care for him in a way too—not physically but in your own way, yes?

Pete: Sort of. When he will need me is when he leaves that life and tries to make sense of it. I'll help with that.

CHAPTER FOUR

PETE VISITS THE OTHER SIDE OF LIFE

O C T O B E R 2 7 , 2 0 1 9

Elizabeth: Hello, all in spirit or partway there.

Pete: Hi, Sis. I am sleeping. My body is sleeping but here I am. I'm feeling time is close for me to leave my old body. I've gotten used to it, but, well, if I can go on without it, I guess I am ready to leave it behind. It hasn't been a great body, but I guess okay. Look how far I've come!

Elizabeth: Yes, you have, Bro—sixty-three years!

Pete: I know it isn't all my doing. I've had the help of all the pills, shots, and surgeries. Without all that, well, I don't know. Then there's all the people that have helped me—Mom, Dad, all of you, Sis, you too. And then everyone here, my adopted home.

Elizabeth: Adopted?

Pete: Well, I didn't choose it at first. I was too little but eventually I did. I feel I've belonged here even though I like visiting other places, like your house, Sis. And traveling too. But I'm done with all that. I sort of travel now but in my thinking, not moving too much. Can't move too much. You know that. Can't talk too much. That's why I like this writing you do which is our talking. But I think I'm ready to say goodbye. Does that sound strange? It does to me. And scary too. But not as scary as it was before. It just seems what will happen whether I want it to or not. So maybe if I think I want it, if I think I'm ready, maybe that's better than being scared and trying to hide from it.

And if I say goodbye, it is sad but at the same time something else too, although the something else is hard to tell. A bit like finishing something I've been working at a long time and the something is complete, is done. I've done my best—well, maybe not all the time, but I have made efforts.

Elizabeth: Bro, you've done well. Marvelous indeed! I'm impressed with how you've lived your life. I'm glad you have been my brother. I have learned much from you—humor and patience, kindness, forbearance. Do you know "forbearance"? If I'm right, it means sort of enduring without complaining. Anyway, I am a better me because of you. Maybe, in some way, when your body is done, you and I can continue to talk like this if you want to.

Pete: Sis, I don't know, but it has been nice. I will say goodbye now and a big goodbye soon.

OCTOBER 29, 2019

Elizabeth: Here I am writing as day ends. I am ready to hear from anyone.

Pete: Hi, Sis, it's Pete, Bigger Pete, if you will. Yes, Pete is quite close now to leaving you, coming here. There isn't much that holds him there, from his point of view. He's already invested so much of himself in what happens next and gets impatient for the next better life. Just keep doing your work and what you do for him. And I thank you, as Bigger Pete, for your care and concern for your brother Pete. Now get some rest. Your bodies need that. Bed bug bite, isn't that it?

Elizabeth: Yes, it is!

OCTOBER 31, 2019

Unidentified voices: Dear Elizabeth, loyal one, caring one, we are here to speak and to answer questions you may have. Do you have questions?

Elizabeth: Well, I do wonder about the relationship between Pete, my brother, and this other voice—Bigger Pete, who says he is Pete plus,

including other lives, a larger or higher self. How should I understand this?

Unidentified voices: What you have said is correct, and it likely is difficult to understand when on Earth in your physical world, where
people are seen as being contained by their bodies, one discrete body
distinct from the next.

You might say their spirit is contained in a smaller part within
and of their body. If you reverse that, you may be able to see how
it works from where we speak. Individual lives are "contained" (not
really but for the moment) by spirit, by a spiritual reality. That is, if
there is a spirit entity known as A, there may be lives, physical, such
as B, C, D, or metaphysical, that are parts of A. Are you following
our explanation so far?

Elizabeth: Yes, I think so.

Unidentified voices: Furthermore, there is more fluidity of all the forms.
And that is probably harder to comprehend. So, Pete's life on Earth, that
is, your brother, is part of a larger spirit entity that you are calling Bigger
Pete. The name is actually rather good. And Pete is not alone in this. It is
a usual experience. What is not usual is that Pete has what is called Down
syndrome, so his mental understanding of something is limited. And now
his thinking is even less capable because he has what is called Alzheimer's
disease, which affects his brain, so his capability as Pete is what you could
call compromised more than usual. Bigger Pete knows most of this, but
Pete has, at best, only an inkling. He hasn't understood the changes his
body has been going through. It makes him frustrated and, for a while,
rather angry. But now he is mostly just tired and resigned to the fact that
he just can't figure it out or change it. When he isn't awake, his mind can
travel, can catch glimpses of the life beyond the one he knows.

You have helped him here, out beyond his usual awake self, as a
companion. He relies on you, knows he can trust you, knows that
you care and are keenly interested in what he's experiencing, that you
are trying to understand it as well, and that's why we come to assist.
Maybe now you can see why we hesitate to name ourselves as if we
were as distinct and discrete bodies as you are. We are not. But we do
care to help, so that's what we say for today.

Elizabeth: Well, voices, thank you immensely! Pete or Bigger Pete, are you available to talk?

Pete: Hello Elizabeth. This is Bigger Pete, as you call me. I am close by both you and Pete, who is sleeping right now. His sleep is restless as he navigates these last days of his life. And let me explain something. Pete has been in his last days for years. When we speak from this world of spirit, as you call it, we don't have time as you know it, so we're a bit foggy when it comes to time—days and years and such—so when we speak of days, they could be much smaller or larger than yours. So, the advice then is <u>not</u> to take such expressions as matching days, years, and such on Earth. Understand?

Elizabeth: Yes.

Pete: So, when it's time for someone to cross over from Earth life to spirit gets hard to pinpoint. It's not just that no one knows or only some people or entities know but that the sense of time is so different. Does that make sense?

Elizabeth: It does. Is this Bigger Pete speaking?

Pete: Well, now, there too, there's a difference. I am Bigger Pete, different from your brother Pete as you see him now, but I also can draw in other entities here to help explain things. So, there you have it—an attempt to explain how the physical and metaphysical worlds differ.

Elizabeth: Yes, I think so. Thank you.

O C T O B E R   3 1 ,   2 0 1 9

Elizabeth: I am ready to hear from anyone, especially Pete or Bigger Pete. Spirits come near.

Pete: Hi, Sis. Hi, hi, hi, Sis, Sis, Sis. Hee hee. I feel good right now. Everything is okay. I'm having a good time.

Elizabeth: That's great, Bro. Where are you? What are you doing?

Pete: Oh, Sis, I don't know where I am, but it is light and free and happy. And I am here just floating around feeling good, like a balloon, a happy balloon.

Elizabeth: Sounds nice, Bro. May I join you?

Pete: You're already here, Sis. You're already here. Isn't it nice?

Elizabeth: I like how you tell it.

This light, free, happy mood was such a delightful respite from the dull grays of the Alzheimer's decline. I remembered not just happy but downright silly moods we had had over the years before Alzheimer's disease came. And Pete, with his delightful sense of humor, had often been the light-hearted one. Once, when we were sitting somberly in the back of a van with family on our way from a funeral, Pete was repeating quietly what sounded like "pubby, pubby, pubby." I asked him what pubby was. Pete, with a straight face but a twinkle in his eye, pulled repeatedly on his lower lip, making a sound like "pubby, pubby, pubby."

Pete: I haven't been as happy as this for a while. I just move about, no trouble. I talk with you, no trouble. I am happy, content. Everything is fine. Everyone is fine. And it's beautiful. Sis?

Elizabeth: Yes, Bro?

Pete: I am full of love, and love is all around me. In and out, I am love. It's all love. It's all beautiful and light and free. And oh, the music!

Elizabeth: The music?

Pete: Yeah, Sis, listen. It's beautiful. It's singing—no, humming—no, I don't know. It's beautiful music. Oh, it's me humming. I am the music. Sis?

Elizabeth: Yes, Bro?

Pete: How can anything, everything, be so beautiful, so perfect, all the time, everywhere perfect?

Elizabeth: I don't know, Bro, but let's enjoy it, yes?

Pete: Oh yes, Sis. Yes and yes and yes. I can stay here forever. It's happy forever. Forever, forever. Sis? Sis, are you here?

Elizabeth: Bro, can you see me?

Pete: Sort of, but you look different. I know it's you. You are here too, and your music. Your music and my music, they like each other, come together, move up and down, move apart. Sis?

Elizabeth: Yes, Bro?

Pete: Is there anything else?

Elizabeth: Why ask?

Pete: I don't really care. It seems it's all here and I'm here and you're here and everyone's here and I am swimming in happy, swimming in peaceful, a beautiful everything. Sis?

Elizabeth: Yes, Bro?

Pete: It feels like a big please and thank you all together. Sis?

Elizabeth: Yes, Bro?

Pete: I don't want to talk. Maybe sing. No, not sing. Just want to see and hear and feel all this around me. Sis?

Elizabeth: Yes, Bro?

Pete: Can you feel it, Sis?

Elizabeth: I can feel what you're telling me.

Pete: Sis, I love you. I love all of this.

Elizabeth: I will go away and see you later, Bro.

Pete: Okay, Sis. Okay, Sis. See you later.

NOVEMBER 2, 2019

Elizabeth: I ask again for whoever wishes to speak.

Pete: Hi, Sis. How are you, Sis? Thank you for coming. I always like to see you, even when I can't say it.

Elizabeth: Why not, Bro?

Pete: You know, Sis. My talking is not good now. I can think of things sometimes, but if I want to say them, I forget how. The ones I say a lot are easier, but even those just hide somewhere and won't come to my mouth or, well, I don't know, Sis. It bothers me, yes, but even the bother, even getting mad, sometimes hides too. So, if I think about it at all—the words or frustration or anything—it doesn't get clear or stay long, and mostly I just let it be. That's just how things are. Things just don't work as they did. Do you remember, Sis, driving in the car when you said sometimes when we get old, our bodies don't work so well?

Elizabeth: Yes, Bro, I remember.

Pete: And you said at least we still have each other, that that will stay the same?

Elizabeth: Yes, Bro, I said that. It's true.

Our long drives together between Pete's place and our house were hours when we could have long talks together or sing our favorite old songs. More recently on such car trips, Pete would tend to drift off into sleep. I was glad he remembered that conversation.

Pete: I'm glad you said that, Sis. My body is older and not so good anymore, but we have each other still.

Elizabeth: Yes, Bro, we still have each other.

Pete: And we can talk like this, so it's like being together.

Elizabeth: Yes, Bro. We aren't close in touching, but we have this talking that is like a hug, isn't it?

Pete: Yes, Sis. I like it. When you come see me, I can't talk much, but this way I can.

Elizabeth: Yes, I'm glad we can do this. And I'm glad that people by you are taking care of you when it gets too hard for you to talk.

Pete: Me too. Sis?

Elizabeth: Yes, Bro?

Pete: Thank you for being my sister.

N O V E M B E R   3 ,   2 0 1 9

Elizabeth: Good morning, those in spirit world and in between here and there. I am ready to write your words.

Pete: Hi, Sis.

Elizabeth: Hi, Bro—how are you?

Pete: Pete is cozy in bed. This is Bigger Pete saying hello, saying good morning to you where you are.

Elizabeth: How are you, Bigger Pete?

Pete: I am fine—busier than usual but that is okay. It is as it should be.

Elizabeth: Do you know I am collecting these conversations to make a book of them?

Pete: Yes, I realize that—a fine project indeed.

Elizabeth: Any advice or suggestions?

Pete: Don't edit. That is, don't change our words. But you can take things out if they don't suit the purposes.

Elizabeth: What would you say is the purpose or purposes?

Pete: Well, it is a record—a reporting of communication. What makes it of interest is the gap between Pete at this point and me, Bigger Pete, as you call me, and how the spirit can negotiate that gap, how you, living and healthy, can speak through the writing to your brother who can't speak much anymore and also to me, Pete's higher self as you call me Bigger Pete. That, I think, would be of interest to many if they can believe such communication is possible.

Elizabeth: Yes, what you are saying is far from what I imagine Pete or maybe even Bigger Pete would tell me, but, well, I just don't really know.

Pete: Fair enough, and I'll say that is better to say—that you don't know—because it opens up room for knowing to come in.

Elizabeth: You do sound very wise indeed. I would like to include everything that you say.

Pete: Well, you decide. Let me say it is very good that you do this writing, these conversations.

Elizabeth: Thank you, Bigger Pete.

Pete: You are welcome, fine sister.

NOVEMBER 6, 2019

Elizabeth: My hand is ready. My heart is open. I am prepared to write.

Pete: Hi, Sis.

Elizabeth: Hi, Bro. What's up?

Pete: Feels like my toes are curling in. Feels like my stomach wants to lie down and sleep.

Elizabeth: Bro, are you sleeping?

Pete: Yeah, Sis, sleeping and dreaming.

November 9, 2019

Elizabeth: Good morning for me, good forever for you in the spirit world (I guess).

Pete: Hi, Sis. When will you come see me?

Elizabeth: This is Saturday. I plan to come in four days so we can go to your bank. We think it would be good to take your money out of your old bank and put it in a new one. Is that okay with you?

Pete: I guess so, Sis. Why?

Elizabeth: Because the new bank is better, is open more hours, closer to where you live. Several reasons, okay?

Pete: Yeah, Sis, that's fine. I'll see you then.

Elizabeth: Bro?

Pete: Yes, Sis?

Elizabeth: One more thing. That is on Wednesday. Then on Thursday, you have a dentist appointment so you can get your teeth fixed. When you fell in your room at night, teeth got knocked out. K will go with you to the dentist. You can fall asleep while he fixes your teeth, and when you wake up, your teeth will be good. That will be much better for you for talking, for eating. And you will look more handsome too. Do you have any questions about that?

Pete: No, Sis. But will you come with me?

Elizabeth: I'll come the day before and do the bank business with you, but K will go with you to the dentist. I will send you hugs from a distance and then telephone to say hello when you are done. Next time after that when I come see you, you'll be even more handsome. Sounds good, yes?

Pete: Yes, Sis. I don't like to go to the dentist.

Elizabeth: Yeah, Bro, a lot of people don't. But you can sleep while the dentist is fixing your teeth, and then it will be done and fine. So that's all.

Pete: Okay, Sis. Thank you for telling me. Thank you for coming to see me. See you soon.

NOVEMBER 9, 2019

Elizabeth: Here I am in cool of evening, hand ready to write. I have two questions. (1) How does a soul or whoever decide when and where it will be born, and (2) how does a soul or whoever decide when and where it will pass on from life? Who makes the decisions? What or who is involved? Oh, one more: What makes prayer effective?

Putty: My dear one, I am ready to open the gate, eager as you are to see what will come in answer to your query.

Unidentified voices: Dear Elizabeth, we come nameless to you in response to your questions. What you ask generally falls into the category of mysteries. But we can say there are a number of factors as to the death question. Genetics plays a part, as does how one lives. One can shorten or lengthen a life by one's daily habits. That much you know. What you are asking is more about the actual time of leaving the body. Who decides that and how? But even there, there is more complication than you might imagine unless one decides to take his or her own life. And even there, there are subtleties and possible complicating factors right up to the last moments.

About being born, this is not just the opposite. It involves usually much thought as to where and when, to whom one is born. We <u>can</u> say that there is some purpose to it all, not just happenstance.

Pete: Hi, Sis. How are you? I am fine, very fine. An okay day, but I like when I can sleep. That is much easier than being awake. I hope you will come see me. If you do, I won't say much. Talk is hard. But we can hug and hug again. That's always good.

Elizabeth: Bro, I have a question.

Pete: Go ahead, Sis.

Elizabeth: When you leave your body, do you care what happens to your clothes and belongings?

Pete: No, Sis, I don't care. I'm not attached to anything. You can give my things to whoever wants them.

Elizabeth: Okay, Bro. Anything else you want to say now?

Pete: No.

Elizabeth: Good night, Bro.

N O V E M B E R   2 1 ,   2 0 1 9

Elizabeth: Here I am late at night but ready with my writing hand and open heart.

Unidentified voices: We are the unidentified voices who wish to support you in your work and also to say we are with you as your brother fades from your life. You will find, dear one, just how much he has been in your thinking, your life. This will mean two things when he goes. You will miss him and find a hole which he and your concern for him have filled so in recent years. That means also you will have time and the freedom to do other things, most of which you do not know now. But also, his leaving will add to your current project for he will contribute, open up other contributions, and you will be adding your own part of the process. And it will have a fine place in the world.

Pete: Hi, Sis. Thank you for coming to see me. I am more and more in my own world, isolated, sometimes scared, but when we talk like this, everything is okay. So, thank you. Sis?

Elizabeth: Yes, Bro?

Pete: I will be leaving my life soon. There is not much I would stay now for. Life is too hard. I don't know what is next, but I have to guess it will be better, much better.

Elizabeth: I think so too, Bro. And when you are ready, go on your way. I will miss you, but I hope we can still talk like this.

So, I would hold your hands, look into your eyes and say, all is well, Bro. If your life is done and you are ready to leave it, I'll say you did a good life, a very good life, and I wish you the best in whatever comes next. So, I'll say goodbye now, but I hope we continue to talk still and then later when you pass on.

Pete: Thank you, Sis.

NOVEMBER 29, 2019

Elizabeth: Here I am, hand ready, heart open to write, to hear from anyone who wishes to speak.

Mom: Hello, dear. Others have things to say.

Elizabeth: How do you know that? Can you see or sense others in spirit? Surely not all—that would be many. How does it work?

Mom: It may be hard to understand, but it operates on love and interest and thought. If I wish to know of others who wish to speak to you and those others wish to be known, I will know of them even if I am not familiar with them. When you call the way you do, those in spirit come, make themselves available, and I, at the least, will know if there are a few or many. Often with you, there are quite a number because you are a trusted and regular receiver of messages. There is a clear sense you are serious, but I don't know or see all the voices, but I know right now others wish to speak so I can say that, and I'll be quiet.

Pete: Hello, Sis, this is the one you call Bigger Pete, Pete's higher self, including other lives lived, but for now, I am not just bigger or higher but Bigger Pete. Your brother is strong, a very strong soul. You are a strong soul too and see that in each other, but now he is not at his best because of his life-long limitations, yes, but mostly because his brain is compromised. It does not work well. He does his best, but he has become accustomed to not being able to do much or understand much or say much. He cannot even be sure of who is around him, what they are saying. He does like to see you, but he is not always in a condition to see you or appreciate that you are there. If he could, he could tell of his travel between that life and beyond, but he cannot.

Pete, when awake, was definitely disappearing from me. Often, he didn't recognize me or realize that I was with him—a contrast to these conversations, when he was asleep, which were a great comfort to me.

The thread to that life grows thinner and thinner. One day or one night, it will break, and he will leave that life to come fully back into his higher self.

Elizabeth: What does all this feel like to you? It is hard to imagine.

Pete: Yes, I'm sure it is. Pete is a part of who I am and he's faltering. I am keenly aware of it but do not feel it in quite the same way that you sense or feel things. The fact that Pete seems not to be in distress is because he can't express it so easily. Partly also, he has resigned himself to his condition, but also, he is becoming more and more like his afterlife higher self which does not feel in the same way. He is strong but his earthly life is fading, and as it does, his afterlife self becomes stronger. So, he does not always feel or feel as strongly the bodily things that would cause him hurt as before.

Elizabeth: But he complains of his feet hurting, stomach hurting, and so forth.

Pete: Yes, he is very much still in his body. Well, not very much but he can still see, sense, feel, and a strong enough hurt will register if not part of his general disease. That is, a passing problem can punctuate, like an exclamation point, the everyday ongoing condition he has become accustomed to. So, I don't feel as he feels but I am well aware of it all. You are kind to ask, but it may be hard for you to understand. I hope these words help.

Elizabeth: Yes, I guess. Thank you.

Pete: Now I want to say one more thing about you. As much as I like your care and concern, it must not take a toll on you. I think it has. Keep in mind your own health, what you need and wish to do apart from Pete. That way too you'll be able to do what you wish to do for Pete much better. So that's all I'll say now.

DECEMBER 1, 2019

Elizabeth: Hello, all you in spirit or halfway into spirit. I open my heart, ready my hand.

Pete: Hi, Sis.

Elizabeth: Is this Pete or Bigger Pete?

Pete: I would say see if you can tell, but that answer itself should be a clue. Pete is fading, ready to leave that life behind, but he does not know, as Pete, how much easier, more wonderful will be his afterlife. He is likely to say later that if he had known, he would like to have left sooner, but, well . . .

Elizabeth: Who decides when he leaves?

Pete: You have asked this before. It is a combination of things that will ultimately decide the end of his life. It is not a single moment but a spectrum, a continuum which he has already embarked on, sometimes closer to the afterlife, sometimes closer to life. He goes back and forth. This is not unusual, but he has been doing it for years. At last, there will be a move to the afterlife, which is conclusive, and he won't reverse and go back. But why should you need to know who decides that or when that last point will come? He is in limbo and quite alone there, although he has glimpses of those in the afterlife and a vague sense of what it feels like to be there. Didn't or don't you have a wee sense of that too?

Elizabeth: Yes, especially when I was in a coma with malaria in Africa.

Pete: Exactly. The line between life and afterlife is much fuzzier and more fluid and changeable than most believe. And what is the point of knowing all this unless it can serve to help others near their end, especially if they are fearful and sad?

DECEMBER 5, 2019

Unidentified voices: Hello, Elizabeth. We come to commend you for your kindness, your efforts. Your brother knows you care, but his own path and its changes preoccupy him now. Yes, he feels isolated, alone, in body and mind, not well. But in spirit, he is okay because of his visiting where he will go next. One day he will decide not to come back to his earthly body and mind, and he'll be okay.

Elizabeth: Is he the one that makes that decision?

Unidentified voices: We have said that the decision involves more than that, but in part, he <u>can</u> decide he is ready to leave.

Elizabeth: And have I been visiting him on the etheric plane when we both are sleeping?

Unidentified voices: Yes, that is correct. You are quite the traveler too, and your meetings with your brother are soothing to him, but you have much life left to live.

Elizabeth: I'm glad to hear that. I am definitely <u>not</u> ready to leave this life yet.

Unidentified voices: No, he is ready, but you are to stay. Nevertheless, he finds comfort in how you have been serving as a guide for him.

Your complaints about memory are related to this. You are so involved with him there that it is crowding your regular memory, so to speak. Also, you have allowed yourself to get tied closely with him and his memory is failing. Yours need not fail, should not fail.

One way to help your own memory is to relinquish more of his path to himself. Pull back, let him go. Of course, do your regular care, but tend to your own life. Let him travel now where he will on his own. He will find guides. He will find welcome, but from others, not you. You may feel that this is wrong, this pulling away you must do. It may feel like abandonment. It isn't. Wish him well on his path, but it is his own <u>without you</u>. And when he goes, you'll have things to do, but then your life will blossom anew. Your body, your mind, your soul—all will flourish beautifully. Allow this to be an incentive for you to leave him alone, and we mean emotionally. Let him go.

Elizabeth: I thought I was doing that.

Unidentified voices: No, you've been quite tied in. So, pray for his safe and easy departure, for his leaving when he is ready. Say and repeat that you wish him well on his own path, which will be beautiful. Even your writing is a help to him, although perhaps hard for you to see. So go into your day. Enjoy, sweet one, enjoy!

DECEMBER 7, 2019

Elizabeth: It is morning. I am writing, my heart open, my hand ready.

Putty: Hello, my dear poet-author, wonder woman, sister-daughter of Earth. I greet you.

Elizabeth: Hello, Putty. Are you teasing me?

Putty: Not really—just a little. I have grown fond of you. Teasing can happen when people care for each other and feel like playing a little. I know you are a serious person but playful is okay.

Anyway, let's see who is here, who wishes to speak other than me, your devoted Putty.

Elizabeth: Would you tell me more about yourself, if not now, then sometime?

Putty: What would you like to know?

Elizabeth: Didn't you have some problems when alive, like what might be called mental issues?

Putty: Well, yes, I would have to say yes, and I think it was because I, like some others, you included, sometimes travel the edge zones between worlds, and that can be treacherous. One must have a solid foundation, a sort of sure-footedness like mountain goats, to be able to negotiate difficult terrain. I mention this because it can be a danger for you as well as a sensitive, intuitive, artistic soul. You need to stay sufficiently grounded, or you fly off.

Elizabeth: And how is all that now for you where you are?

Putty: Oh, you are so kind to ask.

Elizabeth: Well, I guess I have become fond of you too and more curious about your life—that is, what you, not others, would say.

Putty: Well, the thing is, those zones between worlds are rich with all kinds of insights and treasures, so of course, like miners, we want to go looking for them. But now? Well, my dear, where I am is so full of amazing treasures, I need not go looking for them, so my mind is at peace, full of joy, full of love. Does that make sense?

Elizabeth: Yes, the way you explain it. But can you say more about the amazing treasures?

Putty: Yes, for example, all the things a person, a mind, a soul can do without being encumbered by a physical body. Imagine if you could go anywhere at any time just by thinking yourself there, no need to plan, save up money, put in for requisitions, pack a suitcase, buy a ticket, find the airport, endure those cramped, crowded seats, and so on. You get my point. You just go. You might ask, then, is there any purpose to living a physical life in a physical world? Yes, because what a body gives you is a different set of pleasures of sound, of sight, of all that you can feel. But you, in a physical body, still in your mind, can imagine going somewhere without actually going there, so you have a glimpse of what a non-physical soul can do, but I tell you it is not the same. And the ultimate difference is that here where I am, all is love. That, my dear, you have to admit, is different from all the hate and division on Earth, even though there is some love there too.

I think you have come to appreciate your brother Pete in this, for he is capable of quite unselfish love, without complaint, of others. What he complains of is just what his old physical body gives him to complain of. He brings his charming self to the world. He quietly exudes a simple love to those around him, and those around him can receive it if not too wrapped up in his limitations which there are many of now.

Think of your brother as a being of love. See him this way. He sees you this way. He does not want to focus, never has, on what limits him.

While Pete was still in his working years, a van took him and others to and from their jobs. Once, when the van came to pick him up from home, he refused to get in. It took some time to understand what his objection was about. Eventually, what became clear was that when the van arrived at the workplace, the driver parked in the handicapped zone. That disturbed Pete because he didn't consider himself handicapped. So, he just refused to go at all.

He can certainly get frustrated by those limitations. You have seen it. It hasn't been an easy life for him, but it hasn't been bad because he came into a family who could care for him or who could provide for others to care for him. He has touched many in his own way.

You have seen it, been a beneficiary of it. You can thank him as he keeps thanking you. But the thanks are just the superficial recognition of who the two of you are. You have a special bond with him. He knows it. You have been slowly learning it. He does not want you to falter or suffer because of him. But right now, his physical and mental limitations get in the way of his recognizing you and the bond with you. Never mind. Things are going as they will and you both learn and, in your own ways, appreciate each other. That's enough for now.

Elizabeth: Wow, thank you, Putty.

Putty: I have to admit I had some help on that—not all of it just from me. Now, go into your day. Come back soon.

DECEMBER 8, 2019

Elizabeth: Good morning, all in the world of spirit or in-between there and here, like my brother Pete.

Unidentified voices: We come, the unnamed voices who come to you when you call. When you have a question, we do our best to respond, but you, such a dear one, are welcome to come with nothing but intention to make a connection to our world.

Elizabeth: Is it better to have a question, concern, or someone to ask for?

Unidentified voices: Yes, if that is what is in your mind and heart, but if you are willing and open to what words might come, that is all right as well. Now we will wait, pause, just a little, to see if you wish to hear from someone in particular or have a particular concern.

Elizabeth: Thank you. I so like hearing from anyone, recently especially Pete, Bigger Pete. I have my usual concerns, but for the moment, I have no pressing concern.

Unidentified voices: That is fine. Then we will speak. Allow yourself to write.

Elizabeth: Thank you. I am ready.

Unidentified voices: You are a chosen one. No, not in that big dramatic way you might think, but you're indeed chosen to do the work you are doing. What that means is that you have the gifts of writing and other gifts of understanding that allow your work to be successful.

And you have taken up the work, so we have chosen you—those who can do any such choosing—to watch over you and help you in your work.

It means we do what we can while allowing a free life for you to do what _you_ will, choose what _you_ choose. It is a cooperation, but some are not chosen to be helped in exactly the same way because they make no efforts on their side of such cooperation. This is not to be seen as a punishment—more a matter of timing. When what you might call the seen and unseen worlds work together, there is cooperation toward a purpose, but the effort produces little if only one-sided. Does this make sense?

Elizabeth: Yes, it does, and I thank you for the explanation. Now I do have a question.

Unidentified voices: Yes?

Elizabeth: Have my brother Pete and I had other lives together? If so, can you say anything about that that would help the cooperative work now?

Unidentified voices: Oh yes, it is a wonderful question and shows that you are indeed thinking of your brother beyond this one life. You watch out for him, see to his care, and he and his life have allowed you to develop this communication which you, as a writer, can make available to others for _their_ learning.

So, for right now, your two lives are entwined. And yes, you have known each other outside of this one lifetime, but it wouldn't be of much use to you or him to delve into that now. The recognition of that possibility is sufficient for you to consider, and we are glad to hear it because it means a greater recognition on your part of a much larger picture, a larger scheme of things at work, but let's leave it at that, at least for the moment. Now go on with your day.

D E C E M B E R   1 0 ,   2 0 1 9

Elizabeth: I am ready to write. If Pete or Bigger Pete are available, so am I. Or anyone else?

Pete: Hi, Sis—this is Pete sleeping. I am not well, not well at all. I am glad to be able to speak with you. Thank you for listening. Thank you for being such a good sister. Thank you for everything.

Elizabeth: Bro, and I thank you. If you are getting ready to say goodbye, then I give you a big, big hug and say goodbye too. I hope we can continue to talk like this, but maybe it won't be exactly the same. Is there anything you want to tell me now, anything to do or to say to anyone?

Pete: No, Sis. If you want to say anything to anyone from me, just say love.

DECEMBER 12, 2019

Elizabeth: Good morning, all. I surrender my arm and breathe in the cosmos.

Pete: Hi, Sis. Thank you for talking like this with me. It makes me feel good, very good, when I don't feel very good in my body. My body is not working well. It is fading, folding, and I can't think or move well. I am glad people are taking care of me, but they can't do everything. And I can't really thank them for all their help. But I can tell you and you can tell them. Will you tell them thank you from me, Sis?

Elizabeth: Yes, of course. I will do that. What else would you like to say to me now?

Pete: Well, Sis, I don't see you every day, but I know you care, and you are helping me too. You have been helping me for many, many years. My thank you to you would be a huge thank you.

Elizabeth: That's nice, Bro. I am looking for a recliner chair for you now. It is a Christmas present, supposed to be a surprise. But I'm telling you so I can ask if you would like one and what color you would like—blue?

Pete: Oh, Sis, a new chair for me, a comfortable chair, would be nice, very nice. I like blue because it's like Mom's chair. That makes me feel good.

Elizabeth: Bro, do you know Christmas is coming soon?

Pete: I haven't been noticing Christmas, Sis. I like Christmas, but I am sleeping a lot, and Christmas doesn't come into my sleep.

Elizabeth: Well, Bro, that is probably more important now. So, don't worry about chairs or Christmas, just have a good sleep and rest your body and mind.

Pete: Thanks, Sis.

DECEMBER 13, 2019

Elizabeth: I'm feeling mighty low this morning. I'm tired, my knee hurts. I'm feeling old, low, aching. I know things are not desperate, but I don't feel good. I call on whoever wishes to speak.

Putty: Oh, my dear, what can I say? This sounds so familiar. You sound like me, so much like me, and I am sorry. It isn't an easy place to be. You suffer with the hard knocks of Earth and physical life. Have yourself a minimal day. Listen to music you love. Once you express your state and need and ask for help . . .

Elizabeth: Yes, help!

Putty: . . . it will be given. Now be kind to yourself. I'll open the gate.

Elizabeth: Thank you, dear friend, Putty.

Putty: You are welcome, my dear.

Mom: Hello, sweetie. Admit there are some things you cannot do. You cannot see or hear them but so many in the spirit world are cheering you on. If you make a to-do list, keep it short, simple, and just those things you know will help you feel better. We are rooting for you, my dear. I send lots of love. Don't worry about Pete.

Elizabeth: Easier said than done.

DECEMBER 15, 2019

Elizabeth: My heart is open; my hand is ready to write in the protection and wisdom of Divine Light and Love. I welcome Pete, Bigger Pete, or whoever wishes to speak.

Unidentified voices: Hello, Elizabeth. We are the voices of those who watch out for you and others.

Elizabeth: Are you angels?

Unidentified voices: Well, that would require a lecture on the hierarchies and nomenclature, and it isn't necessary now. Think of us as loving guardian spirits. That's enough for now.

Elizabeth: Okay.

Unidentified voices: We see how you are struggling, trying to hold things together, keep on track and not fall apart. Some things will help. First, get enough rest. Also, keep your sense of humor. Keep your tasks simple, few, and doable. That is our advice for now.

Pete: Hi, Sis, it's me—happy to talk with you. I like traveling with you. When I can see you, talk with you. It makes me feel okay, like everything is all right. Sis?

Elizabeth: Yes, Bro?

Pete: I don't know what happens next. I think I am ready to find out. Right now, I am feeling brave and curious. When I am awake, I feel small, bent, tired, and hurt. So hard, everything so hard. But right now, I am fine. I am happy, free. It's so very nice. Sis?

Elizabeth: Yes, Bro?

Pete: You are a good companion.

Elizabeth: Thanks. So are you, Bro. I have a question.

Pete: What, Sis?

Elizabeth: You don't complain or get angry at other people. How do you do that?

Pete: Oh, Sis. I think it is better just to move away if I start getting angry. When I do that, the anger seems to get smaller, and I can think better. I can get angry at things far away where my anger or upset won't make things worse, like when my team is losing. But I do get angry and want to complain.

Pete, being an avid fan of the Philadelphia Eagles football team, liked wearing clothes—shirts, pants, hats, socks, gloves—with Eagles insignia. He took the team's wins and losses seriously. One time he did become so upset at a loss that he slammed his arm against the edge of his table and broke his arm.

But also, I don't think I can do it well or say very well what I want to say so I just think it and try to avoid the situation. I guess that's an answer.

Elizabeth: Yes, it's an excellent answer. Well, Bro, I hope you have very few things to anger you.

Pete: Oh, well, I don't know, Sis. Bed bug bite.

Elizabeth: Yes, bed bug bite, Bro.

answer.

∽ CHAPTER FIVE ∾

A MOVE IS PLANNED

~~~~~~~~~~~~~~~~~~~~~~

D E C E M B E R   1 7 ,   2 0 1 9

Elizabeth: Hello, all. I open my heart and ready my hand to write.

∽☙

Pete: Hello, Elizabeth. This is Bigger Pete, Pete's higher self.

Elizabeth: I don't know how to explain to Pete about this next move
for him, from where he is to a place near me here. Do you have any
suggestions as to how I can make this a comfortable move for him?

> *When Pete was first diagnosed as having Alzheimer's disease, I
> asked the group home director if he could continue to live where
> he had been living. The answer was that it would depend on the
> nature of his decline. However, because where he lived was not a
> registered nursing home, he would have to leave when his need for
> nursing exceeded what the group of group homes could provide. So,
> I began to look for a suitable place that could meet his needs. The
> commute for me to and from Pete's place was five hours, so I was
> also looking for a new place much closer to us in Pennsylvania.*

Pete: Yes, Elizabeth. This is a big move, but it may be that you feel it
more than Pete does. He trusts you, even if it seems he doesn't know
who you are.

> *My visits to Pete were not on a regularly scheduled basis. If I hadn't
> visited for some time, I would plan to go see him. I went to any
> meetings that involved Pete, and if there were any special incidents
> such as falls, unusual behavior, or hospital visits, I would go see him*

or visit him in the hospital. By this time, when I would see Pete usually every few weeks, I never knew whether he would know who I was or not. Pete's disappearing from me like this wasn't easy, but I was anticipating such a possibility. I had seen my mother through the stages of Alzheimer's when she eventually did not recognize me.

I think you can reassure him that he is moving to a new place closer to you, that you want him to live closer to you so you can visit and see him more often.

Also, tell him that in the new place, there are doctors and nurses who will take better care of him, so he doesn't have to go to the hospital so much if he has a problem. Tell him you will bring his favorite things, clothes and so forth, to the new place. Tell him, remind him he is good at making moves like this. He has done it many times before, and each move was to a better place. Let him know about the place with friendly people. Let him know you and he will both be in the adventure together.

If he does not want to go, tell him that the people where he is can't take care of him well now because he needs more care, special care, and so moving will mean his having the special care. And tell him it is closer to you so you can be with him more. You may be surprised that he is more okay with the move than you imagine. But you can talk to him as you are doing with me now when he is asleep.

Even though I wasn't sure Pete always understood me when he was awake, it did seem that what I said to him in these trance conversations carried over in some small way the rest of the time, or so I hoped. But there was also evidence that he did forget some of our trance conversations, too.

DECEMBER 18, 2019

Elizabeth: Good morning. I open my heart and ready my hand to write.

Pete: Hi, Sis. I am here. I am sleeping, but I can talk with you.
Elizabeth: How are you, Bro?

Pete: Okay, I guess, Sis. But things are moving, changing like I am watching a river, but now I'm in the river. It is not wet water but something else. I am not swimming. I guess I am floating, like in the ocean, but I am not wet. The ocean carries me. I don't have to swim but I am moving. Something is moving me. It is not scary. It's nice . . . like a hug, a gentle hug, like love. It holds me and loves me.

Elizabeth: That sounds nice, Bro.

Pete: I can see you, Sis. You are not floating, but I can see. You are beautiful and full of love. It is all love. We are here, you and me. I am floating. You are . . . I don't know. Somehow you are here and keeping me company. Thank you, Sis. I am not afraid. You keep me safe.

Elizabeth: Bro, I want to tell you something. May I?

Pete: Yes, Sis, go ahead.

Elizabeth: Bro, do you know how you have been going to the hospital a lot?

Pete: Yeah, Sis, a lot.

Elizabeth: That is because there are no doctors where you are who can take care of you. And something else. I like to visit you, but you live far from me. Remember how long it is for us to drive from where you live to where I live?

Pete: Yes, Sis, long drive.

Elizabeth: Well, Bro, it would be good, much better, if you could live somewhere nice that is closer to me, a place that has doctors and so I can visit you more and doctors could help you when you need doctor help. So, I have found a place like that. It is much closer to me, and there are doctors close too.

Pete: But, Sis, I am fine here.

Elizabeth: Well, maybe, but you would feel better in this new place. Do you remember all the moves you have made? So many. The last move? You said then that was a good move, maybe the best one. But now it is time to move again, to a place that is even better. Good idea, yes?

Pete: Will you help me?

Elizabeth: Yes, of course, Bro. I can help pack your favorite things— your Eagles clothes, blankets, and things, your pictures, everything you want to have near you, and we'll bring everything to a new place so it looks a lot like your room now.

Pete: Okay, Sis, I guess so.

Elizabeth: You know, Bro, I want to be sure you have the best place to be. When you moved to where you are now, that was the best place to be, but now the people there who help you are having a harder time helping you, so it is not the best place for you now.

Pete: Oh, I didn't know that.

Elizabeth: They like you, the people where you are. They like you very much. They will miss you when you move, but they want you to be in the best place for you.

Pete: Sis, how can I do that, move somewhere else?

Elizabeth: Don't worry, Bro. I will help you. I will pack up your things. You will go in the van like you do on trips to the hospital or elsewhere, and at the new place, I will be with you to help you settle in, just as we did when you moved last time.

Pete: Okay. You'll help me?

Elizabeth: Yes, of course, Bro. And it'll be like a little adventure, but an easy one—one that you can do very well just as you have done your other moves very well.

Pete: Did I? Did I do the other moves well, Sis?

Elizabeth: Yes, you did very well. You were happy making the move. It was different, but it was good, and you did the move very well. And when you move to the new place, I will be able to be with you more, in case you need any help with things, but mostly just to be with you, Bro.

Pete: That's good, Sis. That's good. If you will help me. Sis, I am thinking about it. I can do it.

Elizabeth: Yes, you can. You can do it very well.

Pete: Okay, Sis, thank you. New adventure. New move. I can do that. Yes, I can do that.

Elizabeth: Good, very good, Bro.

DECEMBER 20, 2019

Elizabeth: I greet you all in spirit or halfway there.

Mom: Hello, dear.

Elizabeth: Are you really here, or is this just me writing routine speaking?

Mom: Oh, my dear, yes, I am here, never far, but if the doubts are rising, just put them on a shelf where you can still see them and carry on.

> *My skepticism about these conversations with the dead, with those in the world of spirit, would still pop up from time to time. I continued the writing practice anyway.*

Elizabeth: Okay.

Mom: And Elizabeth, Pete may not be clear about who you are, but he knows in his higher self that you are near, that you care.

> *By this point in his decline, in addition to Pete's not recognizing me, he seemed barely present to himself either.*

Elizabeth: Thanks, Mom.

Pete: Hello, Elizabeth—this is Bigger Pete.

Elizabeth: Okay, hello, but you and Pete sound like two separate people. I don't really understand.

Pete: No, I'm sure it is hard. That is because you are living a physical life where things are in separate physical containers, physical bodies. Imagine no bodies or bodies with very fluid dimensions, edges that are not hard but changing, and it may be easier. Pete and I can be together or separate. There is more merging, blending, separating going on all the time.

Elizabeth: I think I have a glimpse. Your explanation helps.

Pete: Pete—your brother Pete as you know him in a physical body—is pretty much in that old failing body but not entirely. And neither are you. You especially spend much time <u>not</u> limited physically. This has been true for a long time. It means you can understand more of how the metaphysical works and can explain it to others. And you and your brother can meet and talk where you wish, not just on the physical plane.

Elizabeth: Well, that makes sense.

Pete: This writing you are doing—these conversations with your brother—you could call them out-of-body conversations, will be helpful to others for their understanding too.

Elizabeth: Okay.

DECEMBER 22, 2019

Elizabeth: Good morning, all. I ready my hand to write. My right arm is yours.

Pete: Hello, Elizabeth.

Elizabeth: Is this Bigger Pete?

Pete: Yes! How could you tell?

Elizabeth: I wasn't sure—maybe wishful thinking. How are you, and how is Pete?

Pete: Well, you know the situation with your brother—it is a slow, debilitating disease.

Elizabeth: What, in the grand scheme of things, is to be gained from it? Many are suffering—many more will in the future.

Pete: Yes, a good question. Here is what I will say, some borrowed from others. Think about these last years with you and your brother. While his physical self has declined and there has been pain, he has not suffered as much as one might think. Yes, various complaints, but now it is others, like yourself, who fuss over his care. But think for yourself what you have gained during the same time.

Elizabeth: I feel I have come closer in some ways to my brother. I have learned much from his way in the world. I see how little he complains, how he struggles to connect with others and to respond. He hasn't much to give, as some would say, but he gives so much.

Pete: And did you always think so?

Elizabeth: Not at all. I felt a duty toward him but not so much appreciation of him.

Pete: Exactly. The disease happens in the slow way that it does. Many will struggle with it—those who have it and those who care for those who have it. But if one is willing (and this is true everywhere) to be open to learning, opening to see goodness, all that is possible. The disease is not for that purpose, of course. No, not at all, but it does provide an opportunity for those who recognize it as such. So that's all I'll say now.

JANUARY 7, 2020

Elizabeth: Hello, all. I open my heart, ready my hand, and thank any and all who wish to speak.

Pete: Hi, Sis, it's me.

Elizabeth: Hi, Bro—how are you?

Pete: I am okay, Sis. I am sleepy, but I am okay. Some days are better than others.

Elizabeth: I am okay, but I am sleepy too. Bro, when you think about your whole life now that you are older, do you have any special thoughts or new understandings about your life?

Pete: Like what, Sis?

Elizabeth: I don't know—maybe what were the best parts, the best times, what you are proud of, what you are happy you could do, happy for people you have known, or maybe the work you have done.

Pete: Well, Sis, I do think about my life. I don't know if it has been a good or not-so-good one.

Maybe I have lived other lives that were better or worse.

Elizabeth: Did you hope for anything in this life that you haven't done, or been, or seen yet?

Pete: Oh, yes. I think there are many things like that, but my life has been okay. I don't know that I wanted much, so I am not disappointed so far.

Elizabeth: I guess that's good.
Pete: Yes, Sis. What about you?
Elizabeth: I think I'd have to say a lot, but I really need to sleep now.
Pete: Okay, Sis. Have a good sleep. Call me again.
Elizabeth: Okay, Bro.

JANUARY 9, 2020

Elizabeth: It is morning here where I am. I open my heart and ready my hand to write.

Unidentified voices: Hello, dear Elizabeth. We greet you as you wake up to begin your day. We do not have day and night in the world of spirit. Day and night are about living on a physical planet that turns toward or away from a sun.
Elizabeth: Yes, of course.
Unidentified voices: But we have other things to say. There will be changes in your life.
Elizabeth: May I ask what changes?
Unidentified voices: You will see them soon enough. The changes, some of them will affect many. But there will be some personal changes too. So, do all that you do to stay healthy. And if you keep up this communication, we can help you through any changes you might need help with.
Elizabeth: Thank you. I will do my best.

JANUARY 12, 2020

Elizabeth: I am writing because I cannot sleep. I would ask for anyone who wishes to speak.

Pete: Hi, Sis. I am glad to talk with you. Sis?
Elizabeth: Yes, Bro?

Pete: Why is the daytime hard, the nighttime easy?

Elizabeth: Well, Bro, good question. I think your days are hard because your body is old and not working as well. You need help to get dressed, to eat, to move because your body can't do those things easily, but at night your body sleeps. While it is still, your mind can be active, and we can talk like this. Not hard at all. I believe when we don't need our bodies at all, then our souls become stronger, and we leave bodies behind and keep living without them.

Pete: How can that be, Sis?

Elizabeth: I don't know how it works but I believe that it does. And I believe you and I can still talk like this even if we don't live in our old bodies anymore.

Pete: Well, I don't know, Sis.

Elizabeth: I don't know for sure either, but that's what I believe happens, and it sounds okay for me.

Pete: Okay, Sis. It is a good way to think and believe. Sis?

Elizabeth: Yes, Bro?

Pete: Sis, I wonder if people will remember me if I don't have a body, if I don't live in my body.

Elizabeth: Oh, Bro, I think many people will. You are such a kind, charming person, and many people will miss you, not seeing you in your body, but who knows? Maybe they will learn to talk with you like this. And they will have the many beautiful memories of you.

Pete: Thanks, Sis, you are a good Sis.

Elizabeth: Bro?

Pete: Yeah, Sis?

Elizabeth: If you do leave your body behind before I leave my body behind, will you still try to talk with me like this?

Pete: Yes, Sis, I will try. If I can do it, I will do it, Sis.

Elizabeth: Good, thanks, Bro.

Pete: You're welcome, Sis.

J A N U A R Y   2 9 ,   2 0 2 0

Elizabeth: I write again. I open my heart, ready my hand, and thank whoever would speak.

Pete: Hello, Elizabeth. This is Bigger Pete. I am glad to speak with you about your brother Pete.

He is okay. He continues to travel between your world and this one where I am.

Elizabeth: May I ask a question?

Pete: Of course, of course. What is it?

Elizabeth: Did Pete choose the life he has? Did he want to have the disabilities? Our family?

Pete: Of course, you are curious. Normally this is a matter for Pete to be sorting out, as he is doing, but I know he has said that he wishes you to write all this and share it, so I am at liberty to say a few things. Yes, he, at this higher self/soul level, wanted the life he is having. He knew it would not be easy, but he did indeed choose this life and the family you share.

F E B R U A R Y   3 ,   2 0 2 0

Elizabeth: Here I am, heart open, hand ready to write.

Putty: Hello, my dear. It's good you are back. It is good to stay with this writing as much as you can. Now I open the gate as I send you a big hug.

Elizabeth: Thank you, my dear Putty. I have one question. How can I ask for more evidence to help my readers (and me, I admit it) be more trusting of this information?

Putty: Oh, my dear, I know about the trust issues and you've carried on beautifully building it, but as for others, they too will need to develop trust and allow time to prove the worth of these words from the voices beyond.

Elizabeth: Okay, Putty, thanks.

Putty: Now, the gate . . .

Pete: Hello, Sis, this is Pete, Bigger Pete.

Elizabeth: Which one?

Pete: We are not as separate, really, as all that. Pete is part of me, Bigger Pete.

Elizabeth: Oh, I wish I could understand that better.

Pete: You can. Keep doing this writing, this communicating, and you will keep learning.

Elizabeth: Yes, thanks for the encouragement.

Pete: I know that Pete is going to be asked to move. This may be a bigger deal for you than for him. In any case, don't worry. You will have help. Just do what Pete always tells you: Just walk, talk, relax, and take it easy.

Elizabeth: Ohmigosh, does that ever sound nice just now!

Pete: Yes, yes, of course. Let yourself say it over and over. I do not have much else to say now except doing this writing/talking will help you <u>and</u> Pete.

Elizabeth: Does he know he will be moving?

Pete: Well, yes, sort of. You've told him before. He isn't thinking much about the move you are thinking of. He is thinking more about his next move to us in the world of spirit. That interests him, even though he forgets most of it when he is awake.

Elizabeth: Okay, thank you, Bigger Pete.

Pete: You are welcome, very welcome.

FEBRUARY 14, 2020

Elizabeth: Here I am, pencil in hand, heart open to write.

Pete: Hi, Sis, it's me. My body is sleeping, but now I dream and go places wherever it is nice.

Elizabeth: Where are you now, Bro?

Pete: I am sort of floating. I mean I can move without walking. When I am awake, my legs don't work well, but now I can go anywhere and don't really need to use my legs.

Elizabeth: I think I can do that too by imagination.

Pete: No, it's not the same as imagination. Imagination is still in my body. This is me but no body involved.

Elizabeth: How can that be, Bro?

Pete: I don't know, Sis.

Elizabeth: Bro, what can you tell me about what you are seeing and feeling where you are?

Pete: Well, Sis, I'm not in one place. In fact, the floating is really because the places are different. One place is not cut off, different from others. One sort of flows into another without hard edges between. If I want to go somewhere, I pretty much just think myself to that place rather than walking to that place or going in a car or van or plane or something.

Elizabeth: Can you come here where I am in my house in Pennsylvania and see where I am sitting writing to you?

Pete: Well, Sis, I can see you, but you are not really entirely in your house. Yeah, something of you is there, but I am seeing you—something of you but not the whole body of you. Some part or something of you is sort of like me, sort of floating. Are you asleep too? I mean, your body?

Elizabeth: No, not really. I am sort of half-asleep—my body, that is—and my hand holds a yellow pencil, and the pencil is writing fast on a pad of yellow paper, and my body is sitting on the sofa. It's the middle of the night, but I couldn't sleep so I got up and started to write while I was guessing you are sleeping. We have been doing this now for some time, many times.

Pete: Yes, I know, Sis. It's strange. I don't understand, but I like it.

Elizabeth: So do I. And it feels like I am with you when it is harder now to do the long drive to see you when we are both awake.

Pete: Sis?

Elizabeth: Yes, Bro?

Pete: There is so much I do not understand.

Elizabeth: Me too, Bro.

Pete: Really? I thought you know stuff, understand stuff that I never could.

Elizabeth: Well, I know some things. You know some things too—maybe more or better than I do. I think everyone knows a little bit, and then when and if we put our knowings together—that is, tell each other what we know—then we have a bigger, a shared knowing, right?

Pete: Sounds right, Sis.

Elizabeth: Bro, maybe there are some things you know that I don't, and you can tell me. But now I think I will go back to sleep in my body.

Pete: Okay, Sis. Okay, Sis.

FEBRUARY 14, 2020

Elizabeth: Hello, all. I open my hand, surrender my arm to write with two questions in mind.

Putty: Hello, dear woman. What are your two questions?

Elizabeth: 1. I would ask Pete if he remembers when he is awake these conversations we have and the travels he's doing to the afterlife, the world of spirits. What of his dreaming self and higher self as Bigger Pete does he remember when he wakes up?

2. I would ask Mom what her Alzheimer's disease felt like. And how is it like or unlike Pete's experience of Alzheimer's, which has been much longer? Those are my questions.

Putty: Wow, well, big questions, good questions. Let's see if there are any answers.

Mom: Hi, dear. Let's see—you ask about Alzheimer's. It was rough. I didn't mind so very much the forgetting. I did resign myself to that, sort of, after a while. What was harder was I felt myself disappearing along with the memories. That was hard. And I was scared about what would happen next.

FEBRUARY 15, 2020

Elizabeth: Good morning, all. I ready my hand and thank you all. I wish to continue with my questions for you, Mom, about your experience of Alzheimer's and the comparison with Pete's. I'd like to know whether it's a good idea or not to talk with Pete awake about these conversations. Would it help or confuse? Thanks for any guidance.

Mom: Hello, dear. I am right here, happy to try to answer. I'm glad you are curious about my experience. I know you were there, faithful throughout, but you ask how it all was for me. So, let me say now how thankful I am and I was at the time for all your help and attentiveness. Yes, it was hard for you, but you managed . . . beautifully.

As for me, it just felt that I was disappearing, that parts of me were fading or being swallowed up by something I couldn't understand. And I couldn't stop it. I tried. I fought for control but eventually couldn't fight anymore. The disease won. And I died.

> *She died in 2006, having declined for several years with Alzheimer's disease.*

I did what Pete's doing now—started seeing what I could see from where I was. Do you remember how I closed my eyes?

Elizabeth: Yes, I do.

Mom: When I was awake, closing my eyes sometimes let me see the other things that were happening, the other people I was seeing—my mother and others. It became harder to distinguish between my so-called normal waking life and that other strangeness that I was pulled to.

You see, Pete is experiencing something like that. He has little fight left. He goes back and forth between your world and this one. He is watching, wondering, trying to make sense of it all, but he is losing his words. I still had my words. That is a big difference—a very big difference. I could speak, although it didn't make sense, probably sounded nonsensical.

Elizabeth: Yes, sort of. I wanted to understand what you were saying. Some sounded like childhood memories or . . . I don't know.

Mom: But talk connects us. Pete has so little of that, so he developed pet phrases to see him through and his gestures too. But now, even that, those pet phrases and words are vanishing. He feels ever so much more isolated, and here's the thing—it is hard. Why? Because Pete has always been a very social guy, so the isolation is sad and he's lonely. That's why, my dear, your conversations with him now, as you are writing them, is such a blessing, such a relief, so he feels more connected. He craves that, even as he is preparing to leave his life. So, I commend you. Do you remember how I'd try to tell you what I was feeling?

Elizabeth: Yes.

Mom: He cannot do that when he is awake, but when he's asleep, the words are available. When you think about it, it's really a marvel that he manages as well as he does. He is indeed struggling. It's a difficult and strange task to negotiate between where and who he is and what, in his sleeping self, he is remembering as his higher or bigger self. But most will see only his limitations now, not his valiant efforts.

FEBRUARY 15, 2020

Elizabeth: Here I am, ready pencil, to write.

Pete: Hi, Sis, it's me. I am sleeping, dreaming. You are my dream.

Elizabeth: Will you remember talking with me now when you wake up?

Pete: I don't know, Sis. Usually, I do not remember dreams. Or if I remember, I cannot tell about them. Because the dreams are strange, and my words are not working very well.

Elizabeth: Would you like me to talk to you about these conversations when you are awake?

Pete: I don't know, Sis. Why?

Elizabeth: I guess because I know about them when I am awake, and if we don't talk, then it feels like I'm keeping a secret from you. I don't want to keep secrets from you, especially secrets about you.

Pete: Well, Sis, if you have to talk about it, okay, but I am fine whether you talk about this or not. It doesn't feel like keeping secrets from me. Maybe it is too hard to talk about and it's easier not to. I like easier things these days. When I am awake, there is so much that is hard. I cannot think well or talk well or move well. Maybe it's better to keep these conversations for when I am sleeping, and we can talk without real spoken words because I'm not good with words these days.

Elizabeth: Okay, Bro.

FEBRUARY 16, 2020

Elizabeth: I am ready to write.

Pete: Hi, Sis. Sis?

Elizabeth: Yes, Bro?

Pete: What is the point of living?

Elizabeth: Why do you ask?

Pete: I mean, we all die, so what do we get born for? Lives are not so long.

Elizabeth: Yes, well, that's true. I think people get born for different reasons. Some just want to live a life on Earth, feel things like gravity, see things and so forth, or to try to live better than some other life. But I guess it depends on the person. Maybe not a great answer, but that's what I think right now.

Pete: Okay, Sis, thanks.

Elizabeth: What do you think, Bro?

Pete: I'm not sure, but if we were supposed to do something, how do we know what that is and whether we did it or not?

Elizabeth: Oh boy! You've been thinking.

Pete: Well, Sis, I am ready to finish this life, but I don't know if I have done the life right. I don't think so.

Elizabeth: Oh, that's hard, Bro. I don't know. I think one thing that can happen is, after life, you can think about it. For now, you're still living it.

Pete: That's true, Sis. But it feels a little bit like a job, and I can't tell if I have finished the job and if I did it well enough, like keeping the plants in the nursery watered just right.

Elizabeth: Bro, from what I can see, you've done this life well, very well.

Pete: Thanks, Sis.

Elizabeth: I'm planning to see you tomorrow.

Pete: Oh good, Sis. I will be happy to see you.

FEBRUARY 18, 2020

Elizabeth: Hello, all in spirit or in-between.

Pete: Hi, Sis, it's me. Thanks for coming yesterday. I wanted to tell you things, but you know it's just so hard.

Elizabeth: Yes, I know, Bro. Do you want to tell me now when it is easier?

Pete: Yes, Sis. I want to say I am feeling good.

Elizabeth: Bro, I am so glad to hear it. You have a new medicine—Percocet—that helps with the pain. Maybe you are not hurting so much now. Where does it hurt when you do have hurt?

Pete: Well, Sis, my back hurts. Sometimes my stomach. But sometimes, it just starts there and goes out to my legs, too. Then they feel wobbly, or I don't feel them much at all. Sometimes it's like that—not so much hurt, just not so much of any feeling.

Elizabeth: Oh, Bro, why didn't I think to ask you this before? It is hard for you to say about your hurts when you are awake. But you can tell me pretty easily this way. Do you have other things to say about what your body is doing and feeling?

Pete: Sis, my body feels old and tired, but sometimes that just doesn't bother me so much. And I like when I can be strong and free when I am asleep. It's good to sleep. Yes, the rest, but it's also when I can sort things out and think better about everything.

Elizabeth: That sounds good, Bro. Would you want to sleep all day and night if it feels so much better?

Pete: No, not really. I like seeing and being with the people I like, like you, Sis, and doing my regular life, but that other life, when I go places, is really nice, and when I talk like this with you, it's nice, and then I wake up, and there's just so much I can't do. I don't like that. But I like that people care for me. I like that I have a good place to be and I am cared for.

Elizabeth: Yes, Bro, that's good. That's important. Oh, Bro, I hope you can stay where you are for as long as possible.

Pete: Me too. Sis, you are a good sister. I am glad I can talk with you like this.

Elizabeth: Me too, Bro, very glad.

F E B R U A R Y 1 8 , 2 0 2 0

Elizabeth: I am writing to ask for guidance. What to do about the move for Pete?

Mom: Hello, dear. Trust. Have faith. All will be well. Time for Pete to move. He will be okay.

Do what you can. We will do what we can from here to help him and you.

Pete: Hi, Sis. You have told me about the move to the new place. If it is time, that is fine. I am ready. I will miss my friends. It will be different, but I trust you, Sis.

Elizabeth: I will be able to see you more often, Bro.

Pete: Yeah, Sis, you told me. You are scared?

Elizabeth: No.

Pete: About the move?

Elizabeth: No, mostly right now I think I am tired.

Pete: Oh, okay, Sis. I guess I am a little bit scared.

Elizabeth: Well, there will be people helping all along the way.

Pete: That's good, Sis. I need lots of help.

Elizabeth: Me too, Bro. We all need lots of help. And we can help each other. And we will be meeting new people. You are good at that.

Different people will be taking care of you. We will get to know them.

Pete: That sounds okay, if we do it together.

Elizabeth: Yes, Bro. I will be helping and doing all I can.

Pete: I know, Sis. You always do.

FEBRUARY 21, 2020

Elizabeth: Here I am with open heart and ready hand to write.

Pete: Hi, Sis—how is your life?

Elizabeth: Bro, it's okay. I think it will be next week or the week after that you will move. This is a good time to move. Some of the people who take care of you now are moving somewhere else. It will be different for you and me too. But it will be good. Bro?

Pete: Yes, Sis?

Elizabeth: I called you today, but you were sleeping. They told me that last night you were up and about, wheeling down the hall, knocking on doors. Is that right?

Pete had been using a wheelchair for some time by now. Apparently, he managed to get in the wheelchair by himself during the night and wheeled himself out of his room into the hallway of his group home.

Pete: Yeah, Sis. I was looking for someone.

Elizabeth: Who were you looking for, Bro?

Pete: I was looking for my room. Then I was looking for someone. Then I was looking for some other place, but I didn't find anything or anyone. Then I got tired.

Elizabeth: Oh, I see, Bro.

Pete: Well, Sis, if I am leaving, maybe I better get ready and say goodbye to people here.

Elizabeth: Yes, Bro. That's a good idea. I plan to come on Tuesday and help pack your things to go to the new place.

Pete: That's good. Sis?

Elizabeth: Yes, Bro?

Pete: I want to go somewhere.

Elizabeth: Good. When you do move, Bro, I will meet you at your new place where you will have your own room.

Pete: Okay, Sis.

MARCH 2, 2020

Elizabeth: I am ready to write. I surrender my arm and thank all who would speak. I would like any help or guidance about Pete, the coronavirus, politics, anything.

There were the first cases of COVID-19 in the United States by this time.

Putty: Hello, dear. Glad that you're doing this. You can think of this connection you have as your "sanity connection." Yes, you have stress. We wish to help.

Elizabeth: Thank you, Putty.

Putty: Shall I open the gate?

Elizabeth: Yes, please.

Unidentified voices: Hello, Elizabeth. We come to your call with reassurance. All will go well with your brother's move. There are many helping around him—those you know of whom you can see and those you cannot. Keep doing what you do, but yes, take care. Other things are happening that make a high stress level.

Elizabeth: The coronavirus?

Unidentified voices: Yes, that, but we will do our best to protect. Take care of yourself.

Elizabeth: Anything you can say that those of us here on Earth should now know?

Unidentified voices: Well, yes, of course, but for now, we will say simply, keep abreast of news and take care of yourself. Do all your good healthy things to do.

MARCH 3, 2020

Elizabeth: I ready my hand, surrender my arm, and thank all who would speak.

Pete: Hi, Sis, it's Pete—tired, but here I am. Tell me something good, something nice, Sis.

Elizabeth: Well, yes, I can do that. I can say all is ready for you to make your move to a new place. I have told you before. It is a nice place where people will take care of you. You don't know people there. But you will make new friends, as you have done where you are now and everywhere else you go. It will be new, and you will be good at learning the new place. I will be near you. I can spend more time with you because you will be nearer my house. So, we will be doing the new thing together.

Pete: Oh, Sis, I don't know.

Elizabeth: You will do the move well, just as you have done before many times. And many people will be helping you, including me. So even if you don't seem to remember me sometimes, I will be with you, watching out for you, Bro.

> *By this time, Pete never recognized me when we were awake and together, face-to-face. This continued to be difficult for me, but this communication through the writing helped me enormously to still feel in touch and know what was going on with Pete.*

Pete: Good. Sis?

Elizabeth: Yes, Bro?

Pete: Thank you, Sis, for watching out for me. Sometimes I need help.

Elizabeth: Yes. Everyone needs help, so we help each other. Anyway, I am going to sleep now, but I will come see you tomorrow, and next week you will move to a brand-new place. So, nighty-night.

Pete: Bed bug bite, Sis.

MARCH 7, 2020

Elizabeth: I am here with ready hand to write. Any guidance for me? I open to you all.

⌐♾

Putty: Hello, my dear. Let's see who wishes to speak.

Mom: Hello, dear. It's about Pete. He is in the process of saying goodbye to his life there, but he also is building his life here. One thing he has learned is gratitude—and the power of gratitude. He is working out how to show it to all those who look out for him in small ways and large. You are such a key person. He wants to show you the thanks that he feels. He is working out how he can do that. Of course, he tells you, doesn't he?

Elizabeth: Yes, again and again.

Mom: That's not enough for him. He wants to show you in a way much more meaningful, more wonderful, for you.

Elizabeth: Yes, well, not necessary.

Mom: This is not for you to decide. He has this wish, a wonderful one, and all you have to do is receive his gift.

Elizabeth: Wow. Well, okay—my turn to be grateful, I guess.

Mom: Anyway, he wishes to speak, so that's all I'll say now.

Pete: Hi, Sis. Sis?

Elizabeth: Yes, Bro?

Pete: What is it that you want to say?

Elizabeth: I want to say that you will be moving this week to a new place. On Wednesday you will be moving.

Pete: Why, Sis?

Pete, having lost language when awake, was still able and continued communicating through this writing when he was asleep. However, it seemed some of the forgetfulness of Alzheimer's seemed to permeate his sleep state as well. Repeating things and reminding him of previous conversations became more necessary. The repetition in these conversations is evidence of that.

Elizabeth: For one thing, the good people there can take better care of you now. Also, it is nearer to my house, so I can come spend time with you more. It's time for another move. You are very good at moves, and now it's time to make a move again. I will be helping. We'll do it together.

Pete: Okay, Sis. On Wednesday?

Elizabeth: Yes, in a few days from now.

Pete: Okay, Sis. You will help me?

Elizabeth: Yes, Bro. I am packing your clothes, your Eagles things, your picture albums, and such. This is Saturday. I will come on Monday to do more packing. Then on Wednesday, you can go in the wheelchair van to the new place. It is a long ride, like coming to my house. I plan to be there when you arrive to meet you. You will have your own room like you do now.

Pete: I hope my friends can come with me.

Elizabeth: Well, they will not move with you now, but they plan to visit you. Maybe later they'll move there too. For now, it's you that's moving, and I will be helping.

Pete: Okay, Sis. When?

Elizabeth: On Wednesday.

Pete: Okay, Sis. I will be ready on Wednesday. I can do this.

MARCH 8, 2020

Elizabeth: I ready my hand to write and thank whoever would speak about anything (even coronavirus).

Pete: Hello, Elizabeth. This is the one you call Bigger Pete. Please do not try to figure out every little detail. You and your brother are in good hands. Yes, continue to do what needs doing, but relax. Pete may not be happy to move from where he is, but his new place will be fine for the short time he is there.

He is ready to join all of us in spirit. As you know, he has been negotiating the move for years. You can reassure him that he is very good at moves of all kinds. He is a "move expert." He doubts his abilities. He always has. Remember to reassure him how capable he is. And wherever he goes, he makes friends and makes his place his home. Remind him, remind him. He needs this now.

As for you, do what everyone advises. Take care of yourself.

When Pete passes on—I mean the next after this move—he will want to speak with you. Keep up this good work. I don't have any big, dramatic things to say. What you are doing for your brother and this, with your brother, are big and dramatic. Trust me.

Also, I sense you worry about the big virus. Understandable. I will say this: Take all proper precautions. Keep your life simple. We will be doing all we can from here to protect you and your loved ones. Earth and Earth creatures are of a different sort, and we don't wish to meddle, but we do wish to help, especially those like you, doing such fine and important work.

I am glad for this connection and value it enormously. And you, my dear, have yourself developed by leaps and bounds, both through this work and through the attention to your brother.

There is much you cannot see, but luckily, you have learned to trust that which you cannot see.

So, I applaud your work and honor you, Elizabeth.

On Wednesday, March 11, Pete moved into a nursing home as planned. The move went well. There were no major problems.

On Thursday, March 12, the nursing home decided to close its doors to all visitors as a precaution to keep out COVID-19.

So, in spite of the plan for Pete to be closer to family, Pete was now there in a room by himself in the nursing home. No family or friends could visit him. He knew no one there. No one there knew him. And he could no longer speak.

CHAPTER SIX

DISEASE COMES AND
DOORS CLOSE

~~~~~~~~~~~~~~~~

M A R C H   1 3 ,   2 0 2 0

Elizabeth: Help! It is night when I worry more. But at least Pete is safe and being cared for. I'm afraid of the coronavirus—for myself, for my family, my friends, everyone. I am sad and discouraged. I have to say a huge thank you to all who have made Pete's move a success so far. I am so very glad and hope he stays well and content. So, I open my heart and thank you all, whoever you are.

~~~~~

Putty: Oh, my dear, the travails of Earth—you are in them now. I hear your cry and will open the door for those who would speak, who would reassure.

Elizabeth: Thank you, Putty, thank you.

Mom: Hello, dear.

Elizabeth: Oh, Mom, thank you. I'm sure you have had a big part in Pete's successful move so far.

Mom: Yes, well, my dear, pat yourself on the back for your huge part too.

Elizabeth: Thanks, Mom. Maybe though I'm feeling out of the frying pan into the fire with the coronavirus now. I am scared.

Mom: Yes, dear, understandably. And you want me or others to say that you and everyone you love will be spared. Your love for so many makes it hard to give any such guarantee. Of course, I will continue to do what I can (which isn't much) to help. Just because we pass into spirit, that gives us no such powers, but I wish much longer life for you and all the good work you are doing. You have much support. I think you know that. This virus is strong, and many already have suffered because of it. Take good care of yourself.

Pete: Hi, Sis.

Elizabeth: Hi, Bro. How are you?

Pete: I am fine, Sis. I am okay. I know I am seeing many new faces. People are taking care of me. They are kind. They know what to do. Thank you, Sis, for finding a new place for me. You know I cannot do so much now, so I am glad for all the help. And I can sleep and eat and do some new things. It is okay. Really, Sis. I am fine. So, Sis, you should sleep well too now.

Elizabeth: Yes, Bro, I will. I don't know how, but I hope you will tell me if you need anything. If you do, I'll do my best to help.

Pete: Yes, Sis. I know you will. But I am fine, so you can take care of yourself. Stay home, stay quiet. Sis, you will be fine. Don't worry about me.

Elizabeth: I'll try not, Bro. I think I will go to sleep soon.

Pete: Bed bug bite, Sis.

Elizabeth: Bed bug bite.

This conversation was hugely reassuring, given the strange new circumstances of the virus and the impossibility now for any family to visit and see Pete face-to-face.

───────〜〜〜〜〜───────

M A R C H 1 5 , 2 0 2 0

Elizabeth: I ready my hand. Life in a Time of Coronavirus. How might we be of help to others, especially our closest ones? I thank you for any guidance.

───○

Putty: Hello, my dear Earth woman. Yes, you have the troubles that Earthlings have.

Elizabeth: I guess you don't?

Putty: Well, no—think of what worries you—a lot that pertains to physical bodies that are so vulnerable.

Elizabeth: Ah, yes, true.

Putty: But writing as you do this way, in touch with those in spirit, will help you immensely keep things in perspective. From what I see, you're doing well and will continue to do so. You know what to do. And you're doing it. Remember the things that do help physical bodies—rest, simple good food, exercise, quiet time.

You worry about your brother. He is fine. He is okay, being cared for well. No, you can't see him, but trust me. He is doing as well as he can. And people will come to know him and, as you know, take to him. Allow it.

Elizabeth: Okay, Putty. Thank you.

Putty: Now is a good time for your at-home tasks and work. You will come out of this time feeling grand for what you have done and how you've survived. You will do the right things. You will have support. Sure, learn about viruses, but do your own work. It is good work, and people are eager for it. So, after all that, I open the door for whoever would speak.

Unidentified voices: Hello, dear Elizabeth. We are the voices who come nameless to you, to encourage you when things are rough. All this is rough for those who must find a way to work, care for others, keep their sanity. Many will fall one way or the other. It will be a trial in so many ways.

You have us to advise you. We support you and your work, your kindness to others. Of course, we support others, but they may not realize that or don't believe it. These stressful times are hard. As you've seen, one thinks first of oneself and those who one loves, but extend out your caring. Send encouraging thoughts to others who need it. Many do. If you feel a voice, a desperate voice, you may answer with prayer. Your prayers are strong, very strong indeed. Take time each day to devote to those who struggle. Thoughts and words are enough in these days of isolation. We do not wish you to fly around in an effort to help. Younger ones will do that. You can stay home, write, pray, send healing help through thought, through meta-energy. You understand. And all the while, we support you and your work. Be well. You will be.

MARCH 18, 2020

Elizabeth: I am open to whoever wishes to speak. I ready my hand and try to stay awake.

Pete: Hi, Sis. I am in a new place. People, the women, are kind and careful. It is okay. Sis, maybe I won't be here much longer.

Elizabeth: What do you mean, Bro?

Pete: I mean I am in this place, but maybe not for many times.

Elizabeth: Not sure I understand.

Pete: I feel in between here and somewhere else. I am not always really here, not really awake here, not really completely alive here. Sort of in between day and night, awake and asleep, here and there, in between.

Elizabeth: Well, you seem to be doing well where you are. Everyone says you are doing well. I am so glad.

> *Family visits to the nursing home were prohibited because of the virus. Phone calls were allowed, but they were scheduled. One had to wait one's turn. And Pete couldn't speak anyway because he had been losing language. Sometimes he said "Yes" or "No" but could say little else. It seemed he could understand some of what was said to him but not well. So, the gap between any form of conversation when he was awake on the phone and these conversations when he was asleep was huge. When he was awake, there was almost nothing, but in these conversations, he sounded almost normal.*

Pete: I am okay, Sis.

Elizabeth: I'm glad to hear it. Bro, is there anything you might want to tell me now?

Pete: Well, yes, if I could. Maybe many things, but I can't talk well now. It's easier not to talk.

Elizabeth: Well, Bro, even without talking, you seem to be doing well, and the nurses there like you. I like hearing that. I think, "Hooray for Pete!"

Pete: Aw, Sis, you're funny. Hooray, haha!

Elizabeth: Well, Bro, you've done well, very well, so I say hooray.
Pete: Well, thanks. Sis?
Elizabeth: Yes, Bro?
Pete: Where are you, Sis?
Elizabeth: I am in my bed in my house and sort of half-asleep so we can talk like this. It isn't real talking with sound, but our thoughts travel on their own and my hand writes them down.
Pete: That's good, Sis. You can do that?
Elizabeth: Yes, Pete. This is how we have been talking—like thinking to each other across the miles. But I am getting sleepy, so I'll say good night for now.
Pete: That's okay, Sis. Sleep is good. Bed bug bite.
Elizabeth: Yes, Bro, bed bug bite. Until next time.

MARCH 19, 2020

Elizabeth: Here I am, afraid as anyone else. What can anyone say about this virus? What advice, guidance, comfort, can anyone offer? I thank all who would speak, especially are there some ways I can help others?

Putty: Hello. What the people on Earth are experiencing is scary indeed. People will die. Many people. You know the measures to protect yourself. Do them. Encourage others to do so too. I will open the gate for other voices.
Elizabeth: Thank you, Putty.
Putty: I love you, Elizabeth. Let my love surround and protect and comfort you now.
Elizabeth: Wow, Putty. I thank you and don't know what to say.
Putty: Say nothing. Let the love wash over and through you, cleansing and healing and soothing all your frayed nerves.
Elizabeth: Oh, oh, oh . . .
Putty: Now I open the gate.
Mom: Hello, dear—I ache for you. I wish you well, to keep well through these times. It's time for Pete to come to us, and you've helped him

immensely. But it's not time for you. You have many years left and good work and teaching to do. So, take care of yourself now. I send lots of love, oodles of love. There's plenty here, plenty to spare. Spread it around.

Pete: Hi, Sis. Call me and talk to me. I cannot talk, but I can listen. Call me tomorrow. I am thinking of you and how you've helped me. So much help. I want to help you. I will find a way.

And I'll find a way too so that you know the help is from me. But, Sis?

Elizabeth: Yes, Bro?

Pete: I think you want to sleep now, and that is good. You need that now, so sleep as much as you can. I sleep a lot too. When I am awake, everything's hard. Sleep is so nice. You go to sleep, Sis, and see what I mean.

Elizabeth: Well, Bro, you're right. I am ready to sleep. I'll call tomorrow.

M A R C H   2 1 ,   2 0 2 0

Elizabeth: I ready my hand and thank you all.

Elizabeth: Oh, Putty. I am sad and confused in the uncertainty. We all wish to be assured things will be okay. But it's hard.

Putty: Yes, my dear, of course. If I could, I'd lend you my shoulder to cry on. You know whether it's hard for you or not, you feel the suffering of others.

Elizabeth: I think the worst is yet to come. I want to be strong and also a shoulder for others to cry on.

Putty: Yes, my dear. I know that of you. Take care of yourself. You can stay strong for those around you. Mark my words. You will find a way to assist others but not before it is clear, all is clear from the virus. So, build your strength, your faith, and take care. The time will come for you to help. It is not now.

Pete: Hi, Sis—it's me, Pete, going down.

Elizabeth: Hi, Bro. I tried to call you today. No luck. I'll try tomorrow. You don't have to talk.

I'll do the talking.

Pete: Okay, Sis. That's fine.

Elizabeth: I cannot come visit you because the doors are closed to visitors to protect you from a virus. I have been calling to see how you are.

<center>~~~~~~~~~~~~~~~~~~~~~~</center>

M A R C H   2 2 ,   2 0 2 0

Elizabeth: I am open to anyone. This wrinkled hand is at your service.

~⊙

Pete: Hi, Sis. I am fine. How are you?

Elizabeth: For now, I am okay. I send you hugs. I cannot come see you because visitors are not allowed now. There is a disease that spreads easily, so the people by you are protecting you and themselves while they keep taking care of you. So, because the doors are closed right now, many families are calling in, as I have been doing, especially because we cannot come visit while the disease is around.

Pete: Oh, Sis. I guess that is right. Thanks for telling me, Sis. I will do the best I can without your visits.

Elizabeth: Oh, good. Yes, Bro, do the best you can. You can do things well—this too—and I will try to do my best too.

Pete: Sis?

Elizabeth: Yes, Bro?

Pete: Is the disease scary?

Elizabeth: Yes, it is scary. And right now, it is all over, so they tell people to stay home and stay safe. That is what you are doing. That is what I am doing, and that is important. It is a good thing for now. So, take good care of your wonderful self. Rest. Take it easy. And while I cannot visit you, we can talk like this. As long as you and I want to do this, we can talk like this.

Pete: I want to, Sis. Thank you, Sis.

Unidentified voices: Hello, Elizabeth. We are the unidentified voices, as you call us. We are here to commend you for continuing this writing, for your concern for your brother, for your trying your best in this time of stress and widespread death and disease. You know the precautions. Do them. We wish to help in any way we can. This writing you do should help you very much. Organize your days, but that doesn't mean exhausting yourself. When you are well-rested, it will be easier to stand, to withstand the strain.

Elizabeth: Thank you. I appreciate your guidance.

M A R C H   2 4 ,   2 0 2 0

Elizabeth: Good morning, all in spirit or halfway there. I thank you all for your words.

Unidentified voices: We are here, the ones without names. We wish you well. Yes, we do what we can to help but remember, you humans are not the only ones on Earth.

The voices did not mention all the animals here, but of course, changes in the environment can mean changes for all the animals as well.

The Earth is changing, and all that abides on Earth wish, in their own way, to continue to abide. We know you are one who understands that. As a writer, it is good for you to share that with others.

The virus is a reminder, serves as a correction. It will go where it will, and you must protect yourself and continue to remind others not to go overboard—not to be greedy, destructive. This is a time for love, for cooperation.

You think of your brother. He is okay, is in good care. You have done your part and then some. Now, tend to what you can do there where you are. Keep things simple and loving. Now go into your day with our love and support.

Pete: Hi, Sis. I am sleepy, but I want to say hello. Don't worry about me. I am okay. I am meeting new people. People are taking good care of me. Thank you for your help, for finding this place for me. It is good, very good. I like the food here. I like my bed. It does funny movements like in hospital. This is sort of a hospital but feels nicer, more friendly and not so much poking.

Elizabeth: I'm glad to hear that, Bro.
Pete: Take care of yourself, Sis.
Elizabeth: Yes, Bro. I will. You take care of your wonderful self.
Pete: I will, Sis. I love you, Sis. I love you, Sis. I love you, Sis.

MARCH 26, 2020

Elizabeth: I ready my hand, breathe in the cosmos, and thank you all. I want Pete to be okay.

Putty: Hello, dear. Putty says Pete is okay. He is okay and you are okay. He is being taken care of. He knows you care. Maybe he will speak.
Pete: Hi, Sis.
Elizabeth: Hi, Bro—how are you? I cannot visit you. The disease is all around. They have closed the doors so you will be safe and the disease won't get in. I can't visit you, but I send my love to you, Bro. While you are sleeping, receive my love, Bro. I'm sleepy too. You are safe where you are. I am safe here where I am in my house. I will try again tomorrow to call you, but if you are asleep, that's okay. You need your rest. I know they are taking good care of you, but right now, I cannot see you so that both of us can be safe. So, take good care of your wonderful self. Bro, are you okay?
Pete: Yes, Sis. I am fine. Don't worry about me. We can talk like this even if you cannot visit me. You are a good sis.
Elizabeth: You are a good bro. Sleep well, Bro. We'll talk again.

MARCH 27, 2020

Elizabeth: I open my heart. I send love to Pete and hope I can speak with him now.

Pete: Hi, Sis—this is me. Sis?
Elizabeth: Yes, Bro?

Pete: Things are different. Around me is changing. I am changing. I'm not sure what is happening.

Elizabeth: Well, what is happening is that you are in your new place. You left your old place. The people there are taking care of you—helping you to shower, get dressed, eat meals, take your meds, make sure you are comfortable. I think they are doing that well, aren't they?

Pete: It's okay, Sis.

Elizabeth: That's good. I know it's different from where you knew everyone and everyone knew you. But when you first moved to your old place, you didn't know people and they didn't know you, but you made friends and you can do the same again. You don't have to do anything special. Just be your wonderful self. You are already making one or two friends, I think, yes? People like you. So, you're doing great. You did the move very well indeed. And now you're learning the new place. And from what I hear, you're doing everything very well. Hooray for you!

Just keep being your wonderful self. Now, because of the disease that's around, maybe you will have to eat in your room or do activities in your room for now. And I cannot visit you, but when the disease goes away, I can. That might be a long time, but we can always talk like this. It's not the same as being together, but I can sort of visit you this way. And you can tell me whatever you want to say, okay?

Pete: Okay, Sis.

Elizabeth: Okay, that's good, Bro. You are safe. I am safe. I love you, Bro.

Pete: I love you too, Sis. You are a good sis. Bed bug bite.

Elizabeth: Bed bug bite, Bro.

Pete: Elizabeth, this is Bigger Pete. Get ready. Pete is getting ready to leave that life. So, you should get ready too—whatever you have or want to do. Give him permission and let go.

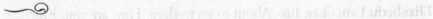

MARCH 28, 2020

Elizabeth: I open my heart, ready my hand, and thank all who would speak and those who remain silent in spirit.

Pete: Hi, Sis—I am here. Thank you for talking with me today.

Elizabeth: I was glad to hear your voice, that you are okay. I am glad.

Pete: I am okay, Sis. I know you cannot visit me now, but do not worry. I am okay, really.

Elizabeth: That's good. Do you have anything to tell me, to say to me now?

Pete: No, Sis. I am fine as I am. I have had a good life. I am ready to leave.

Elizabeth: Well, Bro, when you leave, I will miss you, but do not stay for me. You have done very well. There is nothing you need to do now. That is good.

Pete: Sis?

Elizabeth: Yes, Bro?

Pete: When I leave this life, will you leave too?

Elizabeth: No, Bro—I hope to stay here for more years to finish the work I need to do. I hope if you go first that we can still talk like this after you've gone. You can tell me all about where you go and what you see.

Pete: Good night.

MARCH 30, 2020

Elizabeth: I am ready to write. I thank whoever would speak.

Unidentified voices: We come to speak. You have raised up your everyday energy by an act of will. Not easy, we realize. Do have confidence that you will see this crisis through. Yes, do all you need to do for protection. This will be a bit of quiet for you. Cherish it. It won't last forever.

Elizabeth: Good things or bad things coming?

Unidentified voices: Let's say that it won't be as quiet or you as retiring. That's all.

Pete: Hi, it's me. How are you, Sis?

Elizabeth: I am okay, Bro. About to go to sleep. How are you, Bro?

Pete: Sis, I don't have much of a life now, mostly sleeping. It's very quiet here. I need help with things.

Elizabeth: Yes, with a lot of things, I know, but people are there to help you.

Pete: Yes, Sis, but they're far away.

Elizabeth: Bro, do you know that you can call them?

Pete: I can't talk well, Sis.

Elizabeth: That's okay, Bro. You have by your bed a button on a cord. If you push the button, it rings somewhere else, and someone will hear and come to see what you need.

Pete: Like in hospital.

Elizabeth: Yes, exactly. Where you live now is a little bit like a hospital with nurses and doctors.

Pete: Sis?

Elizabeth: Yes, Bro?

Pete: I don't know about the button.

Elizabeth: Bro, shall I call and ask one of the nurses to show you?

Pete: Yes, Sis, please.

Elizabeth: Okay, Bro, I'll do that tomorrow.

Pete: Thanks, Sis. Sis? When can I see you?

Elizabeth: I can't come visit, Bro, because there is a bad disease around and so, for now, visitors from outside cannot come visit. When the disease goes away, I plan to come visit again, but I don't know yet when that will be.

Pete: Okay, Sis. Sis, are you sleepy?

Elizabeth: Yes.

Pete: Well, go to sleep. Bed bug bite.

Elizabeth: Bed bug bite.

A P R I L   5 ,   2 0 2 0

Elizabeth: Hello. I wish to write and thank you all—those who speak, those who are silent.

Mom: Hello, dear daughter. I thank you. You have more than fulfilled my wishes for Pete's care.

  This snag at this end is universal indeed—not your doing.

Pete: Hi, Sis. Thank you, Sis. I am glad you are my sister. If you can call me, that would be nice. If you cannot, that is okay. I can say this to you now. I want to say goodbye. I am ready to leave this life. I know you will stay. I hope we can still talk like this. We will see. I know that I want to, now as I think of it. You too, yes?

Elizabeth: Oh, yes, if we can. Anyway, you have been a good brother. I've learned much from you.

Pete: Sis?

Elizabeth: Yes, Bro?

Pete: I love you and I trust you to decide things for me.

Elizabeth: Thank you, Bro.

Pete: If you want to sleep now, go to sleep. We don't need to talk, but I always like it. Now you have a good rest, Sis.

Elizabeth: Thanks, Bro. You too.

<center>~~~~~~~~~~</center>

A P R I L 1 0 , 2 0 2 0

Elizabeth: Hello, all. I am ready.

Pete: Hi, Sis. I'm going.

Elizabeth: Going?

Pete: I'm leaving, Sis.

Elizabeth: Bro, I will miss you. Many will miss you. So many love you, but I hope you and I can still talk. There is Bigger Pete—your bigger, higher self—who holds your hand and mine. See, we can stand together holding hands in a circle. I'll let you go on your way with lots of love. I will stay here. You are the brave explorer, like a knight in shiny armor questing. Before you go, is there something you wish to know that I could tell you or find out for you?

Pete: Well, Sis. I want to know if I will be okay.

Elizabeth: Yes, Bro, you will be fine. You may be sad at leaving this life that you've done so well, but you can cross to the next life. You can do the crossing well, and you will do the next very well as you've done with this life. You will be free, happy, and you won't need any of the armor. The armor is like your body. It is old and tired and doesn't work so well now. You know you can't walk well, talk well, and do all the things you used to do. You can now leave that old body behind. You will still be you—the important part of you. You will be free and happy. And Bro, I hope when you do leave and get to know better where you are going, please let's still talk together. I won't go with you now where you are going. I have work to do here, so I will stay, but I will come later so I'll see you again then. But you go first, and I will come later. You are like a grand knight on a horse pursuing your adventure. Do you understand what I am saying?

Pete: I think so, Sis. It sounds okay.

Elizabeth: Yes, it'll be better than okay. And you can tell me all about it.

Pete: Okay, Sis. Sis?

Elizabeth: Yes, Bro?

Pete: I will miss you. I will miss this life.

Elizabeth: Yes, but it is getting too hard to do this life now, so now is a good time to leave and go somewhere new.

Pete: Okay, Sis.

Elizabeth: Where you are now, the people there, the women, the men, the nurses and doctors, they're taking care of you. Now they wear masks on their faces to protect you and themselves from disease. It looks funny, but it is okay.

Pete: Oh, okay, Sis. Sis?

Elizabeth: Yes, Bro?

Pete: Sis, what will you do when I go?

Elizabeth: I will cry. I will miss you. But then I'll get all these conversations we've had, make them into a book for others to read, as you have said I should. So, when people read, they'll remember you and what a fine person you are. Some time we will have a gathering of people who love you. We'll sing songs and remember you and wish you well wherever you are.

Pete: That sounds good, Sis.

Elizabeth: Yes, I think so. I hope so. Do you have any questions that I might answer?

Pete: Yes, Sis. You are very smart. I'm not so smart. Why?

Elizabeth: Well, Bro. You have had a disease. It's called Alzheimer's disease. It makes you less smart, and it makes it so you don't want to talk. Just sleep. Mom had that disease too and then she passed on. You can join her when you leave this life. I'll say goodbye now, but I hope to talk with you later.

Pete: Okay, Sis. Okay, Sis.

APRIL 12, 2020

Elizabeth: Here I am wishing to write and thank you all. I am happy to hear from anyone.

Putty: Hello, dear. We capture you into our surround of love, you who have done well for your brother. I know—we all know—he is about to leave you and come join us here. Rest assured—he will be fine. He will be free, happy, and well-loved. I will open the gate.

Mom: Hello, dear. Yes, Pete is on his way here. He comes well-loved. I thank you for all you've done with him, far exceeding the promise I exacted from you.

Elizabeth: Oh, Mom, I am so glad he's been my brother. I am so glad for all you did. He is so dear, so amazing, so incredible. I wish him a safe, easy journey to you.

Mom: We will do all we can to ease his way, and he will be welcomed with such love that I don't think you can imagine. Maybe Pete would speak now.

Pete: Hi, Sis.

Elizabeth: Hi, Bro. What can I say? Most important: I love you. I am so glad you've been my brother. You are an amazing person, and when you leave this life, I will miss you.

Pete: I'm leaving, Sis.

Elizabeth: Bro, yes, you leave when you are ready. I cannot come give you a goodbye hug. The doors are closed to all visitors because there is the bad disease outside. They are protecting you. We are staying safe in our house. We'll be okay where we are. But we wanted to come say hello, so we came yesterday and waved at the window, but we couldn't come in to give you a hug. That is why we stood outside your window. The nurse moved your bed close to the window. I don't think you could see us, but we could see you. The nurse opened the window so you could hear us. I don't think you could tell where our voices were coming from.

Pete was lying in a hospital-like bed. He had an oxygen mask on. When I spoke to him through the barely-opened window, I could see that he grabbed the bed rail and tried to pull himself up but couldn't quite tell where my voice was coming from. His arm looked so thin. He must have lost weight in the mere month he had been in the nursing home.

That's okay. Bro, I know you could hear us saying we love you.

Pete: I love you too, Sis. You are a good Sis.

Elizabeth: Now you're about to leave us, but I hope you and I can still talk like this, not in words aloud but in our thoughts back and forth. Bro, I say goodbye for now. We all wish you well, our wonderful brother. Soon you will be free of disease and struggle. You will be leaving to go to that beautiful place with Mom and Dad and others. They are waiting for you, ready to welcome you when you are ready, so I want to tell you that. No reason to be afraid. Everyone loves you, and you will soon discover the life after life. You will be fine—more than fine—happy, free.

So, I say goodbye, Bro, as you leave this life. Maybe you are sad to leave this life—and everyone you know and love. I can understand that. And all of us will be sad when you do leave.

But we all say go when you are ready. We all wish you well. Do you understand?

Pete: Yes, Sis, I do. I am okay. I know you're okay. Thank you for coming close, for coming to my window. I am beginning to be something different, something more than I was, something more than the brother you know. My body is changing. Some of it is shutting down, turning off, not working.

But something else is happening, Sis. It's like a big, lovely wave that comes to buoy me up, like loving arms that carry me. It is so strange, Sis. But I'm not afraid. It's as if love is a person or a big friendly animal or just a big, round, bouncing ball of happiness and okay. Sis, I don't know if I can tell it well. You are the writer. You tell the story.

Elizabeth: Bro, you are telling it better than I could. You are a poet, and this is your experience.

You are opening up to a brand new different but beautiful life.

Pete: Sis, I am leaving Pete. I am leaving myself.

Elizabeth: Are you afraid?

Pete: Not at all, Sis. I am just watching and listening and feeling the light and the swirls of light and color. I am okay. I am just going, letting it happen. It is beautiful. I am leaving myself. I am leaving Pete and Pete's body. I am becoming Pete but more than just Pete. I am becoming strong and gentle and beautiful and fine. I have no pain. I have no struggle. Everything's easy.

Everything's easy. I can do this. I am doing this. I am doing it well. I am strong and I'm smart.

Sis, I am smart. I know that I'm smart. I can feel that I am smart. Oh, such a nice feeling. And more than smart. I'm becoming wise, a very wise man, and more than that. Sis, I am a wise and very loving man and, Sis, guess what! I'm not just a man, but I can be a woman too. How can this be? Sis, this is amazing. How can I tell it?

Elizabeth: You're telling it, Bro, and you're telling it beautifully! Oh, Bro, you are smart, and you are wise, and you are loving. You have always been loving, your whole life long.

Pete: Oh, Sis, I don't know if I can say more now. I don't want to report. I just want to do this, and if I can, I'll tell you later. I know you will listen and tell this story. So, I say goodbye to you, to Pete, to all those and this life. It has sometimes been hard. Well, it's time to go. Say goodbye to everyone for me. And Sis, a big, big hug for you. I hope we can talk later, but I must go now. Goodbye, goodbye. Love, love, love, love, love, love, love . . .

Elizabeth: Here I am ready to write in the protection and wisdom of Divine Light and Love. I open my heart, surrender my arm, breathe in the cosmos, and thank you all, silent or speaking. I dedicate this to Pete as he is on the threshold of life and death.

Pete: Hi, Sis.

Elizabeth: Hello, Bro, can we talk?

Pete: Yes, Sis, we can talk. I am still here but not totally. So much of me has left my body as Pete. I might not recognize you if you were in front of me. It seems I can talk with you, but things are changing. I don't know if I can keep doing this.

Elizabeth: That's okay, Bro. We'll do what we can if you wish to continue.

Pete: Yes, Sis. Yes!

Elizabeth: Bro, you asked me a question before, and I answered it but not completely. I'd like to answer it more now.

Pete: Sure, Sis, go ahead.

Elizabeth: You asked me why you weren't smart.

Pete: Oh, I am getting smart, Sis.

Elizabeth: Yes, I believe that. What I said before was that you have something called Alzheimer's disease. Little by little, it makes memory worse and makes a person less smart, not able to think or talk well. You had it some as you got older. Mom did too. So, you could think better, you were smarter when you were younger before that disease. But there's something else too.

Pete: What, Sis? What else?

Elizabeth: Well, Bro, all of your life, not just at the end, you have had Down syndrome. Some people call that a disability because people that have Down syndrome are less smart than other people. That is why when you were ten years old, you left Rochester, where we all grew up, and moved to the New Jersey school to live because that school helps people with Down syndrome learn to be smarter. I think you never liked that you had Down syndrome because you never wanted even to talk about it. Is that right?

Pete: Maybe.

Elizabeth: Is it okay if you and I talk about that now?

Pete: Yes, Sis, it's okay.

Elizabeth: Do you know what I'm talking about?

Pete: Yes, Sis, I know, but you're right. I don't like talking about it. I was always trying to pretend that wasn't about me.

Elizabeth: Well, Bro, I can understand that because people can be unkind. They can be mean, some people, to people with Down syndrome, right?

Pete: Right, Sis.

Elizabeth: But that's usually because they don't understand about Down syndrome, so they act mean, which is not at all a very smart thing to do. It would be smarter to try to learn.

Pete: Sis?

Elizabeth: Yes, Bro?

Pete: You are right. I know I was different, and I didn't like it, so I tried to ignore it, but it didn't go away.

Elizabeth: Yes, I can understand. Down syndrome happens for all of a person's life, but that person can decide how to think and act about it. I guess you decided to try to ignore it. In fact, I think you and I never really talked about it. And you have had a good life, an amazing life anyway. And something else, Bro . . .

Pete: What, Sis?

Elizabeth: You are smarter than many people in several ways.

Pete: How, Sis? How am I smarter?

Elizabeth: You are more kind than many people who think they are smarter. You bring joy to people. That is a wonderful thing. You have been an amazing guy, even if you haven't been as smart as some other people supposedly are. I have learned a lot from you.

Pete: Like what, Sis?

Elizabeth: Like the fact that you take people and things as they are. If you don't like someone or something, you just move away. That is much smarter than being mean or nasty or arguing. Also, you hardly ever complain, even when times get rough, or you find things hard to do. And you are so kind and loving. I have seen all that and admired it and tried to be more like that myself.

Pete: Wow, Sis, I didn't know that.

Elizabeth: Well, Bro, I guess it's about time I said it. And something else, Bro. I don't know why you came into the life with Down syndrome, but you made a good life anyway. I believe when you leave, the Down syndrome part will stay with your old body and you won't take it with you.

Pete: Oh, Sis, I think that's right. I've started to leave that old body, and I can be and do things that my old body couldn't do.

Elizabeth: Well, that sounds good, Bro. I hope your life after life will be wonderful and you will be as strong and gentle and smart as you want to be. I hope you will continue to be as loving as you are now and always have been because that's the most important, and at that, you're a whiz.

So maybe that is more of an answer about your smart question, okay?

Pete: Yeah, Sis, thank you. I'm glad you said all that.

Elizabeth: Good. Now that we've talked about that, I'm going to go to sleep. I'm guessing you are already asleep. And Bro, again, don't stay in your old body for me. I'll miss you, but I'll be glad for you when you go on, leave this life for a more beautiful one. So, I say goodbye now to Pete, to my wonderful, smart, amazing brother Pete. And I hope we talk again when you are in your life after life.

Pete: Okay, Sis. Sounds good. Thank you, Sis.

Pete passed away from life on April 15, 2020 at 11:53 P.M.

OBITUARY

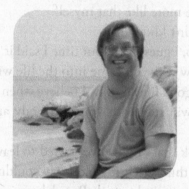

August 4, 1956 – April 15, 2020

Peter Ward Taylor, who preferred being called "Pete," was born in Rochester, New York, the youngest of five children. He was the son of the late Thomas Curtiss Taylor of Rochester, New York, and the late Charlotte Little Taylor of Winona, Minnesota, who lived many years in Rochester and then Princeton, New Jersey, before her passing.

Pete lived in Rochester until the age of ten, when he went to the Bancroft School in Haddonfield, New Jersey. He spent a number of summers at the Bancroft facilities in Owl's Head, Maine, which he enjoyed very much. He participated in various work opportunities offered through Bancroft. He particularly liked greenhouse work but also did clerical work and other jobs. He had a "second family" at Bancroft, where he nurtured friendships with staff and other persons served for more than fifty years. He lived in Dogwood House at the Flicker Residences in Voorhees, New Jersey, until his move to the Pennsylvania nursing home just a month before his passing.

Pete was always very fond of popular music and dancing, and also sports, especially the Philadelphia Eagles. He enjoyed trips to the Adirondack Mountains, Minnesota, California, and Cape Cod, as well as to east Africa and the Holy Lands.

In his life, Pete faced several challenges, mostly associated with Down syndrome and also the devastations of Alzheimer's disease at the end of his life. Nevertheless, Pete, a great hugger, had an affable, fun-loving personality and enjoyed times together with family and friends, including friends at Bancroft. He brought joy to many. One of his favorite expressions was, "all is possible, all is possible."

PART II

AFTERLIFE

CHAPTER SEVEN

GONE FROM EARTH, WELCOMED ELSEWHERE

A P R I L   1 6 ,   2 0 2 0

Elizabeth: Here I am, ready to write and thank whoever wishes to speak.

Putty: Hello, dear woman—you want to see who is here, ready to talk. Fine, I'll open the gate.

Elizabeth: Thank you, Putty. It's starting to sink in about Pete being gone.

Putty: Ah, yes, well, you'll see he may become more available to you now.

Elizabeth: I am patient.

Mom: Hello, dear.

Elizabeth: Oh, Mom, what is happening with Pete? Where is he? What is he doing, seeing? What is the process of crossing over? Can you tell me? Is Pete doing it well? He was so worried he wouldn't.

Mom: Hello, dear—don't worry. All is well. You may laugh at this, but you must remember how Pete likes a good party, especially if it is all about him. And he's having one now.

Pete did indeed like a good party. Three years before, for his sixtieth birthday, he had arranged, with much help from those at the group home, a birthday party to which all thirty-six residents and staff were invited. He requested that all men wear something with the insignia of his favorite football team—the Philadelphia Eagles. And the party décor was all about the Eagles. He asked that the women dress in black. When I asked why, he said, "Because it looks good."

He's the star of his own welcoming party. He has been visiting for years, and there's quite a throng to meet him and greet him and make him welcome. No, he doesn't need his body. He's fine without that old thing. He can't talk to you now. He is indeed busy, but I expect before long that he'll want to tell you all about it.

The process? Not the same for everyone, depends on the person, what they want, what they need, all sorts of things. Your brother is practically a celebrity, and he's already loving it. Don't be sad for him.

And something else, the conditions were not great at the end of his life. You were shut out, but, dear, he needed that to finally relinquish and release that life. It's possible to hold people past when they're ready to go. He's crossing just fine. He's doing it well, very well, and he knows it. I'm enjoying it too. It's so great to see him, to see his struggles over and to see his rewards for the life he has led. The biggest reward is release from that old body. It's a glorious feeling, even if the dying body isn't much of a shackle.

Now, dear, tend to Pete's things and then enjoy. Oh, how you helped me and then Pete. Time for you to enjoy *your* life. So, keep checking in. Before long, Pete will talk. I'm sure of it. But now, dear, you must rest—a well-deserved rest. That's all from me. Love from your mother.

A P R I L   1 9 ,   2 0 2 0

Elizabeth: I am here, ready to write. I dedicate this to my brother Pete and to Bigger Pete.

Mom: Hi, dear daughter. You are still helping Pete.
Elizabeth: Yes.
Mom: His obituary and such. Now take time and relax.
Elizabeth: It's hard. The waves of sadness. It's there, the grief, like a power, a presence that just envelops me, steps in when it pleases.

Mom: Yes, well . . .

Elizabeth: Is Pete available to talk yet?

Mom: No, I don't think so, but you can ask.

Elizabeth: How?

Mom: Just ask.

Elizabeth: Okay, Pete, are you there? Can you talk?
[Pause]

Mom: It's all right, dear. Your rest may be more important now. Try to sleep.

Elizabeth: Okay, Mom.

A P R I L   2 0 ,   2 0 2 0

Elizabeth: Here I am. I open my heart. Pete, can you talk? I am waiting . . .

Mom: Hello, dear. Pete's doing fine. I know you're not. Grief comes unbidden, even when you don't think you feel any grief.

Elizabeth: True. As if a cloud just settled on me, a cloud with its own wishes and plans, all unknown to me. Mom, can Pete talk yet?

Mom: I don't think so, dear. It may be a while. There's just so much going on. He is being celebrated, and he is trying to fathom just who he is, who he was, where he is, and so forth. For someone like Pete, this may take some time.

Elizabeth: Why?

Mom: Because the life he took on was so fraught with challenges. He was so limited, and he knew it, but all on his own, he did it beautifully. And I have to say, Elizabeth, you helped enormously. You always have been an advocate for him, and he knows it.

So, he is trying to figure out that life, this place, what happened at the end, and what will happen now—a lot. He may send messages through others or just check on you to be sure you are okay. He knows how hard that ending was for you as well as for himself. Certainly not what you expected.

Elizabeth: No.

Mom: But it may have hurried him here, and there's no harm now because he is here and well-welcomed. Sis, as he calls you, you did a good job. He may not call you that now. He will be finding his way back to his own higher self—the one you call Bigger Pete (good name). But as you wish to hear from him and he is quite busy, why don't you rest and try again later.

Elizabeth: Thanks, Mom.

APRIL 22, 2020

Elizabeth: I know I'm distracted but also dreamy, so I hope this is a good time for this.

Putty: Yes, dear, this is Putty. You are an adept after all these years. You just need to ask, to state your wish and intention with gratitude. We are here, much closer than most people imagine. Let's open the door.

Unidentified voices: We come again as unidentified voices. We come to say about your brother in spirit. He is being welcomed and is busy with that.

Elizabeth: My eyes are watering.

Unidentified voices: Keep going—it's okay. It'll stop. Your brother Peter is doing fine. He has been welcomed warmly by those he has known from this past life—your mother, father, sister, and others—and by those who knew him from elsewhere.

Elizabeth: Elsewhere?

Unidentified voices: Your brother is an unusual spirit—a very brave one. If souls were a quantity, his would be overflowing. He takes on a lot for himself to endure for several reasons. It helps him to learn, it relieves such enduring hardships by others, and well, he has his own agenda.

Some here have called him Christ-like for how much he loves others. You may find this strange. We are not inventing this to please your ears. Not at all. You don't need or want that.

You want the truth. We know that of you. So does your brother.

You two have much together in your lives in various capacities. It is not at all strange you were born into the same family. There is no way either of you bring this knowledge into this lifetime consciously. You both wanted to live this life as you have, but little by little, you both came to see, to feel, a bond you could not consciously spell out, and at the same time, there has been a recognition of your strong karmic, some might say, connection. Let it be. It's nothing you must do anything special about.

Both of you have been doing beautifully—on your own and together. He was reluctant to leave you. It is good you kept saying it was okay for him to leave. And his not being able to see you, your not being able to visit, was actually a boon for his earlier departure—not any earlier than intended.

The fact that Pete moved into the nursing home and then the very next day, due to the virus, the doors closed to visitors was exceedingly difficult for me. I had arranged for him to move away from his familiar home where he had lived for so many years to a strange place where he knew no one and no one knew him. To make matters worse, he had lost language. He couldn't stay where he had been living. He needed the nursing care. Also, the nursing home was much closer to me. I had been counting on visiting him regularly, and now I couldn't visit at all. It felt as if I had abandoned him. The guilt I was feeling was enormous.

You have plenty, you and this brother, to busy yourself with. All that you've written with him, about him, may be shared widely. You have yet to learn of the marvel of your brother, but you both are amazing. And we give a blessing to your efforts. So, take care of yourself and get on with the work. Yes, you are a writer. Write! Then later, when your brother speaks with you, you and he can decide how you wish to proceed. Oh, and yes, we are doing what we can to help you through the scourge. You do your part.

Elizabeth: Thank you, dear ones. I'll do my best.

<hr>

APRIL 22, 2020

Elizabeth: I open my heart. I hope to hear from Pete. I'm feeling quite devastated. My eyes are heavy.

Putty: Hello, dear one. Yes, it is hard, very hard to lose one you love, one you have responsibility for. Let's open the gate.

Mom: Hello, dear.

Elizabeth: What is Pete like, in spirit? How do you recognize him and he you? Is he glad to see you, you to see him? I'm having a hard time with his going. I'm feeling lost and dazed.

Mom: Oh, dear, I am so sorry. Yes, I am glad to see him. Of course, he isn't in his Earth body, but, well, he is my son. I know him. I can explain maybe but perhaps better later. Not important now. Dear, Pete is okay.

Elizabeth: Yes, you told me, but this overwhelming feeling is not something I seek out. It comes and takes over . . . just like that when it wants to.

Mom: Why don't you speak to your grief like a writer? Tell what you're telling me. Tell it to the grief. Pete will want to talk, but not just yet. Better for you to rest and get used to his being gone. And get used to not fussing about him. You did what you could.

Elizabeth: Mom, what can I do now? What matters?

Mom: Oh, dear, you will be sad, overwhelmed, go through the days like a zombie. You'll forget things, get angry, get sad, but you will laugh too. You will see flowers as if for the first time.

Elizabeth: I did, today!

Mom: Yes, and little by little, grief will grow fainter. You'll feel more like yourself. Maybe a different new self. Maybe just maybe you'll take on something of Pete—his loving nature. You have a head start, as kind as you are. But now sleep. Rest will help the grieving. Some things we have to endure, to live through.

Elizabeth: Mom, I don't know. I want to talk with Pete. I want *him* to tell me he's okay.

Mom: Yes, I know. It will come. Go to sleep now. Think of a lullaby.

APRIL 23, 2020

Elizabeth: Here I am. Pete, Bigger Pete, others?

Mom: Hello, dear. Pete <u>will</u> be in touch when he is ready. He has a lot to deal with now, even though he has been visiting here. All that visiting helps, but it's not the same thing. You will see when you come, when it is your time to come. Not yet. You know that. I will be quiet, let others speak.

Unidentified voices: Hello, dear daughter Elizabeth. We know you wish to hear from your brother. Be patient. We will say again for you to get back to your writing. This will help you immensely to move along in your grief. Yes, there is grief, even if you know your brother is fine. He's a big part of you and he's gone. You also are a big part of him. He is busy with other things now, but he misses you too. As soon as he is able, he will want to speak with you. Allow him now his own welcome, his own work in leaving that world and coming here. Much is involved.

APRIL 25, 2020

Elizabeth: Here I am. I open my heart.

Unidentified voices: Hello, dear daughter of Earth. We are here to console you, support you.

You have come to visit as much as you can while still in an Earth body. When you sleep, you take off and travel. You know to come back to your body in your bed. You do not desire to leave Earth as yet. That is as it should be. Your brother has come first. He would like you to come, but you've already told him that you'll remain there for now. Once he feels like speaking with you, he'll feel better too.

He misses you but knows he is where he should be. You both have released what your lives were meant to accomplish in terms of each other.

APRIL 29, 2020

Elizabeth: I open my heart and thank whoever would speak. Is it too soon to hear from Pete, Bigger Pete? I am here. I am sad.

Putty: Hello, dear one. This is your old friend, Putty, wishing to console you. It is not just the passing of your brother that troubles you. You feel the weight of the times—the sickness, the despair, the hopelessness of many, and not just the humans but many of Earth's creatures. But let's do this writing. I'll open the gate.

Mom: Hello, dear . . . feeling a sadness for you and all who suffer. Those of us here wish you well.

It may be soon for Pete to speak with you. He has not forgotten you. Not at all. He is seeing new things, having new realizations, including the bond you have with him. Your bond, your support, your caring buoys him now in this world of spirit that is strange to him but at the same time feels so like home. He is glad to be here. He is not sad. He is grateful for what efforts you made for him. He will tell you himself when he can do so.

For now, take care of yourself. There will be upheavals in your world. Keep your own life as simple as possible. Develop good habits, and keep them in honor of Pete, be as loving as possible. That is most needed.

Unidentified voices: Hello, granddaughter of Earth, angel in disguise.

Elizabeth: I don't feel like any kind of angel at all. I feel on edge. I feel selfish. I worry. I falter. I want to crawl in a hole and go to sleep, then wake up and find the horror is over. Whatever happened to happy, to joy?

Unidentified voices: Oh, dear, these are the voices that come to console you. You are fine but now walking in darkness. But there are gifts of darkness, and you will be given them. You will lie low and reflect, give thanks, and be loving. So, this may not be the voice you were hoping to hear, but go on with things with trust and patience. Love is all around you.

~~~~~~~~~~~~~~~~~~~~~~~~~~~~~

M A Y   2 ,   2 0 2 0

Elizabeth: Hello, all.

Mom: Hello, sweetie. Do you have a question?

Elizabeth: Yes, if you do not have bodies, how do you see and hear, and how do you recognize someone who is bodiless?

Mom: Of course, you would ask this, as I did too. It is a shift. For those of us accustomed to a physical world, we take that as the given, the way to encounter anyone or anything. But think for a moment how you know those you know now. Is it only the physical? No, that makes it easy. But imagine Pete, for example, in his body as you know it. Now imagine the same body but of someone mean and selfish. You would say, what happened to Pete? That isn't Pete. You know him most easily by outward appearance but certainly not only that. I can recognize Pete now without his old body.

Elizabeth: How about voices?

Mom: Not with sound and all the physical voice "equipment." We can think what we wish to say to someone, as I am doing now with you, right? You don't hear my physical Earth voice.

Elizabeth: No, but I do not hear sound. Your words show up on my paper because my arm writes them but not because I am hearing their sound.

Mom: You see? The senses make some things easier, but the world of spirit is not a physical world. It is metaphysical—even beyond metaphysical.

Elizabeth: I guess I sort of knew that.

Mom: How is the grief?

Elizabeth: Oh, Mom, sometimes almost absent, sometimes almost debilitating. I seem on the edge of tears, ready to cry at the slightest thing. I know it will lessen with time. At least I hope so. It doesn't seem to matter that the departing person is in a "better place." Grief seems to function on rules of its own.

Mom: Oh, dear, I'll just say keep love in your heart, and if you can imagine it, think not that love is contained in your heart but rather that you and all are living in the heart of love.

MAY 2, 2020

Elizabeth: I write and thank whoever would speak.

Unidentified voices: We come but with little to say except to rest, be gentle with yourself. Go slow and deep. You will emerge from this well, but it will take time. This is quiet deep time as if you have entered into the deep heart of stone.

MAY 5, 2020

Elizabeth: Here I am. I open my heart.

Mom: Hello, dear. Imagine my being the mother of you both—so different in your lives and such a bond. Thank you for all your help for him.

Elizabeth: It started out as duty, our promise to you, obligation to Peter, but then his magic began to work on me too—an amazing brother.

Mom: Yes, you could see it and others too. I'm glad that you were able to allow that something special to develop, a recognition of the bond the two of you had already.

Elizabeth: Mom, I didn't realize how much of my life he was.

Mom: Ah, yes. Well, you did so much that he was always present in your mind, whether consciously or not. You will discover what you can do now that he has come here and left you there.

Elizabeth: No emergency calls, no unplanned trips . . .

Mom: So much, so much. Now you can rest. This is a good time to rest.

Elizabeth: Mom, what about this virus? Can you say anything?

Mom: Oh, dear, so much depends on how you all on Earth deal with it. It may provide lessons, good lessons, but at the cost of many lives. I know you will be careful. You will find your way.

Elizabeth: Mom, I don't know what to do in these waves of sadness. I feel useless, hopeless, totally I don't know what.

Mom: It's grief, dear—a function of how much your mind, your emotions, your plans—so much has been involved with Pete. Now all that is changed, not all gone but changed. Take care of yourself.

M A Y 6 , 2 0 2 0

Elizabeth: I write. I open my heart. Surprise me!

Putty: Hello, dear wonder woman in this sad time. Stay your wonder self—you are a wonder self. Be calm, expect little, be nicely, lightly surprised at little. All will be well. Trust that all will be well. I have been sad, so sad, so depressed. It is definitely a bummer, to use an old word. I have been there. No fun. We don't wish this on you. Yes, some is grief. Some is the times, the disease. You will be okay. Don't expect much. Just one foot in front of the other. Keep things simple. I'll open the door.

Unidentified voices: We come, the voices without names. We shower you with love. These times are hard—yes, hard. We come to comfort you. Carry on as you have been doing. This will be rough. Many are suffering. You are one who can feel it. You suffer with them without intent. You share their despair, their sorrow, their grief on top of your own. We do not bring surprises. You don't need surprises now, however nice. You need to rest. Rest and remember how this time is. It won't always be. Things will get better. Spirits will lift. That's all we have. Just our attempt at solace—no surprises, just love.

~~~~~~~~~~~~~~~~~~~~~~~~~~~~~

M A Y 2 1 , 2 0 2 0

Elizabeth: Here I am at last, ready to write.

Mom: Hello, sweetie. This is your mother. As for Pete, he is okay. And dear, you are not at fault for your arrangements for him. The move allowed him to say goodbye to everything familiar, and that includes his familiar body, and that also includes you, my dear. You were the steady thing. He knew that, but, well, he'll tell you when he can.

Elizabeth: I am eager to hear from him. I don't want him to think I was abandoning him. It feels like that now.

Mom: Oh, no, dear, not at all. But I know you want to hear that from him.

~~~~~~~~~~~~~~~~~~~~~~~~~~~~~

J U N E 1 1 , 2 0 2 0

Elizabeth: Here I am, hand ready to write. You all know who I would be pleased to hear from, but let me be grateful to anyone who wishes to speak with me.

Putty: Oh, my dear, you're having a hard morning. I hope those beyond, including myself, can help ease your sadness, your sorrows. Just write. Allow those voices to speak through your pencil.

Mom: Hello, sweetie. It hurts to see you suffering. I believe you have many years left, and they will be your best because you will be doing what you like to do—being between two worlds, so to speak, writing and helping others. Your brother Pete is so inclined. He wants to help others. I believe he will do that when he is able.

Unidentified voices: Hello, dear Elizabeth. We are the voices, the voices unnamed. You, dear, are an exceptional soul. This time has been rough for you. This time has been rough for many on Earth. It is important to meditate daily. Walking is good to think and reflect. It's good you are doing that.

Now, about your brother—he <u>will</u> speak with you. He knows you
are eager to hear from him. He is glad others have told you that, so
he need not feel rushed. When you do hear from him, it may surprise you. It's likely to be different from the Pete you know, as your
brother. It is good you have this time to be able yourself to relinquish
him, the him that is Pete. He will be Pete in part but, oh, so much
more. So, we hope this helps.

~~~~~~~~~~~~~~~~~~~~~~~~~~~~~~~~~~~~~

J U N E   1 6 ,   2 0 2 0

Elizabeth: I am ready to write. I am doing this now to see if it helps me
remember all the things I learned from Pete.

—◎

Elizabeth: What have I learned from Pete? He never was at all self-dep-
recating. He had, it seemed, a fine view of himself. I don't think he
ever found fault with himself. I don't think he saw flaws except that he
wasn't as smart as he liked, but he didn't complain. Born under the sign
of Leo, he did seem to have such a sunny, even kingly, disposition. He
did have depression. He had periods of great depression, such as after
our mother died, but it was sadness at the loss, not a poor opinion of
himself. And whenever that depression was with him, he just retreated,
didn't participate in things. I guess he tried his best to sort things out
on his own, maybe not always successfully. Such low spells tended to
last for quite a while, but what he mulled over, what he felt, how he
sorted things out, he kept to himself, probably because it was hard to
explain how he felt. I don't remember ever his feeling sorry for himself.
I have learned from Pete's responsiveness to people. He might or
might not listen, depending on the situation and how much he was
capable of participating, but I never heard him tell people to shut
up or go away. If he didn't want to listen, respond, or participate, he
would just move away, and in later years, his wheelchair years, when
it was too hard to move, he would just tune out.
He rarely complained, even if he had plenty he could have complained about, especially concerning others. About himself, he either

had a very high threshold of pain or just chose not to complain, even when he had a number of issues.

One time, when he was young and our mother was rushing to get him dressed, she accidentally turned one of his toes backward in his shoe. He said nothing. It was only later when he was noticeably limping that someone thought to check his feet.

Late in his life, he had much physical distress that he could have complained about, but the level of discomfort would have to get pretty high before he would moan or groan. He did occasionally moan or groan but seemingly involuntarily. Even when he was asked if something hurt or something was bothering him, he often just said, "I'm okay."

He asked for little, except maybe for a beer or seconds at meals. He had preferences when it came to clothes. A fan of the Philadelphia Eagles football team, he liked wearing Eagles T-shirts, gloves, and so forth, but he was never covetous about clothes, fancy clothes, and so forth. If asked what he might want for his birthday or Christmas, his typical answer was simply, "Something good, something nice." He enjoyed opening presents but never seemed to take unusual or long-lasting pleasure in what gift he might find inside. He wasn't interested in money, hardly ever handled it. Because of his limitations, others typically took care of such things for him. He had no interest in money, getting much, having much, or in collecting what money could buy. Good lesson there!

He was willing to try some new things, which, given his limitations, was significant. Not all things, but he surprised me at times when he would say yes. For example, he would occasionally try new foods. I remember when I tried to see if he would want to write poetry. He tried, wrote a couple poems, and then that was enough. Not his thing. Actually, he didn't write them—he dictated them to me.

I have learned about gratitude from his example. He not only was appreciative of people's efforts, but when he was able, he said so. There are many instances of this. The interesting thing about gratitude (in my experience—he doesn't say this) is that if you decide to be grateful, you then often discover things to be grateful for.

He was patient about a number of things, including about what he couldn't do. He would try again. He would say to himself quietly, "Try again. Try again." His speech was not clear. Those of us who knew him usually understood him, but when we or others didn't, he kept trying to say what he wanted to say. When he learned to spell, that helped. I also learned that talk helps a lot but that it isn't always as necessary as we might think.

Also, by his example, I have learned the importance of trust. All along, he trusted me, and that level of trust does something quite wonderful to elevate relationships, encourages one to act so as to be worthy of trust, for example. Closely connected to the issue of trust is the importance of taking people seriously. I have witnessed that this happens less when people with disabilities may not be taken as seriously as they should be. Also related to this is the issue of where and from whom one can learn.

The issue of learning itself is a huge one. Some people are designated teachers, but learning can happen from anyone, anywhere. When we were growing up, our parents stressed our having always to teach Pete and help Pete because he would need all the extra care and teaching. I didn't see at the time how <u>he</u> might teach <u>me</u>. And I suspect that is the case as many people mistakenly think that it is only those who are said to have a disability who need the help with learning, not the other way around.

Perhaps one of the biggest lessons I have learned was not from anything he consciously taught but in his nature as a very loving person. He loved unconditionally; no strings attached. When, over the years, I was able to relax my obeisance to duty as his sister, I began to appreciate what a kind and loving man he was. I admired that about him.

J U L Y 1 , 2 0 2 0

Elizabeth: I am happy, delighted, to hear from anyone about anything now.

Putty: Hello, dear one.

Elizabeth: Hello. Do you not tire of helping me as gatekeeper?

Putty: No, not at all. For one thing, I do not tire, not having a physical body, and secondly, what or who shows up at the gate is so interesting. So, I am happy to be available.

Elizabeth: But what if you're busy with something else?

Putty: Now, that would be harder to explain. But let me say time isn't the same in the world of spirit, and everything is more fluid. The physical laws of Earth don't apply. You'll see when you come.

Elizabeth: Well, your explanation helps.

Putty: Good.

J U L Y 9 , 2 0 2 0

Elizabeth: Here I am, this time with a candle. I am happy to speak with anyone.

Putty: Hello, dear one—Putty here. I like the candle. It has a magic all its own, as *you* do. I'll open the door.

Elizabeth: Thank you, Putty. Somehow, I feel Pete near or perhaps Bigger Pete, but perhaps it's just wishful thinking by me.

Unidentified voices: No, not wishful thinking alone. We see your brother wishes to communicate with you, but this is a different mode than what you had with him. Then you were both in the flesh but in mind in a slightly altered state.

Now you are still in flesh in the dense physical world of Earth, and your brother is totally in spirit. He is fine, happy, curious, and he knows you wish to hear from him. His attempts to reach you may take the form of signs which you may or may not recognize as such. We know you are trying to be patient and that's good. He knows you can be patient as you have been for years with him. So, carry on in your wonderful way. All is well.

Elizabeth: Thank you (whoever you are).

AUGUST 22, 2020

Elizabeth: I open my heart and thank you all—those who speak and those who support those who speak.

⟫

Unidentified voices: We come, dear soul, right away to support and console you. Now, we want to tell you: trust us, please, this is true—your brother is with us. He is in good hands, learning and remembering what it is to be here as he is now. He is an old soul, a magnificent soul. He took on quite a life and stayed the course of that life for so many Earth years. In that life, he could not see, could not remember the whole picture of himself as he can again now. He was frustrated by his limitations, of course, but, well, he lived out that life and brought joy to many.

He knows you want to hear from him. He is not purposely holding back. Instead, he is working to regain his ability to communicate with you now across the life-afterlife divide. He is happy to have us explain to you what is going on now for him.

You will hear, meanwhile, from others, like us, about your brother. We can give you one strong message from him for you. Do not feel bad or guilty or anxious for the last month of his life. You are not to blame at all for his death. You must not take that on yourself at all. Instead, he wants to thank you in the most eloquent, the most wonderful way that he can, that he is grateful for all that you did do for him. You were one big reason for his wanting to live, to continue that difficult life. He will tell you all this. We are telling you now. He has engaged us to tell you what we are telling you. He will be able to tell you all this himself eventually.

Meanwhile, he is doing all he is capable of doing to help and protect you now in your life. He is aware, vaguely aware of the troubles now in your world. He doesn't want you to be troubled. Instead, you can thank him for his part in supporting you, which he is doing now at the same time as he is tending to what he is doing now for himself and his bigger self. He says you called him Bigger Pete. Yes. So be glad, be thankful. Take all the precautions in order, at this time, to stay safe and healthy, including staying at home, and you will sail through all this. Keep your focus on your work, your tasks, your wonderful husband. Do not be distracted. You have much support. Honor it by doing what you know best to do.

As for your brother, rest assured he does not blame you. On the contrary, he would and does shower all the blessings it is in his power to muster on you and yours. We say farewell for now.

Elizabeth: Thank you, and thank you, Pete, thank you, hugs, love! Yes!

AUGUST 27, 2020

Elizabeth: I write. I open my heart and thank you all.

Unidentified voices: Dear Elizabeth, you might call us the host of heaven—voices from those who care about you, your life, your world. There are many who support you and your work. This is, as you've realized, a retreat time for yourself—involuntary, yes, but one you can use to good benefit.

Elizabeth: May I ask a question?

Unidentified voices: Of course, yes.

Elizabeth: Can you or anyone else tell me the details of what Pete is doing, going through now? Is it like an orientation? Is he learning things? Doing a life review? Meeting those in spirit he has known? Has he made any attempts himself to communicate with me? If so, how? Any advice for me as to how to be receptive? How is he doing? Are he and Bigger Pete, his "higher self," now one and the same? Is what I am asking available for me to know?

Unidentified voices: Whoa there! That's a good deal more than one question and will involve a number of entities to try to answer. Let's see if we can help a bit now. Then this will take some time.

Elizabeth: Okay, thank you.

Unidentified voices: Taking your last question first, some of what you have asked is available for you to know, to learn, but you must realize that Spirit, the world of Spirit, as you call it, operates so differently from the Earthly life you know, that even if you were given information, you would have a hard time making sense. It's not about the words but what the words refer to. One example: You are in a physical body, and the laws of a physical world mean that you must pay attention to those limitations. The idea of an etheric body—even though there are the words—is unfamiliar to you and hard for you to fathom, but we know you wish to learn and are serious about this, so we will do our best to explain. You can also read what others have already written.

And for now, we can say your brother is fine. He is eagerly and energetically learning.

We will say more later. Enough for now. Go into your day. Go in peace.

⤔ CHAPTER EIGHT ⤖

PETE SPEAKS FROM THE
OTHER SIDE OF LIFE

SEPTEMBER 3, 2020

Elizabeth: Here I am, ready to write. I open my heart and thank you all.

Putty: Hello, dear—you are sad. I can feel it. Let's see what happens when we open the door.

Elizabeth: Thank you, Putty.

Mom: Hello, dear.

Elizabeth: Hello, Mom. Was that you in the "corner" of the reading with the medium?

> *I awoke one morning with a name—one I had not heard before. When I searched online to see if there was a real person by that name anywhere, I discovered that indeed there was someone with that name and that she was a medium. I found a phone number for her, called her, and made an appointment for a reading. In the reading, the medium made contact with Pete and our mother and father, among others. Here my mother helped to explain some of what came through the reading.*

Mom: Your father and Pete really wanted to connect with you, so I stayed back.

Elizabeth: Mom, I'm feeling quite lost, don't know what to do. The pandemic, the politics, and Pete gone, and can't he talk now?

Mom: Oh, my dear, yes, he can talk. Couldn't you tell he was so eager to talk? So many were—your father, me, Pete, others. When he learns how to hear you calling and learns how to answer, and when he settles down, he'll speak with you. Give him credit for trying so hard to connect. As he said, don't be mad. Be patient. You can always ask us about him. We're all rooting for you and send that healing blanket of love. Good night, darling daughter. Sweet dreams.

SEPTEMBER 4, 2020

Elizabeth: Here I am to write. Pete, I've wanted to talk with you, but maybe you're not ready to do that now. That's okay. I light the candle with love to all from very spacey me.

Mom: Hello, dear. Stay on track. If you go off, don't go far. Pull yourself back.

Elizabeth: I feel sad, depressed, not sure if I want to keep living.

Mom: This is the result of the extended time shut away and, of course, Pete's leaving. But he is here, and he is fine. So, don't worry about him.

Elizabeth: Okay, I hear you. I'll try.

Pete: Sis?

Elizabeth: Yes, Bro. Is that you?!

Pete: I can't talk well—don't know how to do this.

Elizabeth: You're doing it, Bro! You're talking and I'm writing your words just as we did before you left this world and went off where you are now.

Pete: Sis?

Elizabeth: Yes, Bro?

Pete: Can you hear me, Sis?

Elizabeth: Yes, Bro. My hand hears you and is writing what you say. How are you, my dear sweet Bro?

Pete: I am fine, Sis—happy, free. I can go anywhere, do anything.

Elizabeth: Really? Wow! Is this really you, Bro? Pete? I can hardly believe it.

Pete: Yes, Sis. It's me.

Elizabeth: Are you really fine?

Pete: Yes, Sis. When you come here, you'll see. I can see Mom, Dad, so many.

Elizabeth: I've been missing you, Bro. I've missed you so much. I couldn't work on the book about you and me. Maybe now I can.

Pete: Sis?

Elizabeth: Yes, Bro?

Pete: Can we talk this way as we did before?

Elizabeth: We're doing it, Bro! We're doing it! Hooray! If you just talk to me, I may not hear you, but if I call you by writing to you, you can answer me, and I'll write your words. Then I can hear what you say.

Pete: Anytime?

Elizabeth: Almost anytime. Oh, I am happy. I have been wanting to talk with you. I am so sorry I couldn't be with you on your last days when you were in that new place. Remember?

Pete: I got sick, Sis.

Elizabeth: Yes, that's true. And I'm sorry. But I think you are happy and healthy now, so that's better, isn't it? You had a good, long life, but it was getting harder at the end, especially when you couldn't talk well.

Pete: True, Sis.

Elizabeth: I'm going to stop now, but I will call on you later, okay?

Pete: Okay, Sis.

Elizabeth: If you don't hear me or are busy or don't want to talk, that's okay. I'll just try again later.

Pete: Oh, okay, sounds good, Sis.

Elizabeth: Then I will say goodbye for now and talk with you later.

Pete: Okay, Sis. Until later. Bed bug bite.

Elizabeth: Bro, I miss you.

Pete: I miss you too, Sis, but I'm glad we can talk.

Elizabeth: So am I. So am I.

SEPTEMBER 4, 2020

Elizabeth: I am writing again. Pete, Bro, are you there? I am calling. Can you talk to me? This is night here now. I am getting ready for bed. If you talk to me, I cannot hear you with my ears, but somehow my hand can hear you and my hand can write words you say to me. Can we try it again, Bro? Possible? I send love, Bro, and I hope you can talk to me, yes? I hope so.

———&

Pete: Sis!

Elizabeth: Yes, Bro, you are there! And can you talk with me?

Pete: Yes, Sis! I can talk with you. Mom and Dad showed me how to do this.

Elizabeth: Oh, Bro, I can hardly believe it. I am so happy. How are you?

Pete: I'm fine, Sis. I am happy. I feel good. I feel free.

Elizabeth: Where are you, Bro?

Pete: I don't know the name for it.

Elizabeth: That's okay. Can you tell me about you and where you are now, Bro?

Pete: Sure, Sis.

Elizabeth: How is your body? You aren't sick anymore, are you?

Pete: No, Sis. I am fine. Everything is fine.

Elizabeth: So, you are with Mom and Dad?

Pete: Yes. They are here. They have been helping me. It is different here, Sis. It is very nice. I can go wherever I want whenever I want to go. No wheelchair, Sis. My legs work just fine, Sis.

Elizabeth: Oh, Bro, I am so glad. You sound healthy and happy. What does it look like where you are?

Pete: Oh, so hard to tell, but it is very light and free and pretty.

Elizabeth: Are there lakes and rivers?

Pete: Well, sort of, but you don't really get wet in them.

Elizabeth: Wow, that's different.

Pete: Yeah, Sis. And Sis?

Elizabeth: What, Bro?

Pete: I can be by myself if I want, but people are so nice, and animals are here too, but they are friendly too, not scary.

In his life, Pete was never fond of animals and shied away from them. He didn't even like stuffed animals that were intended as toys.

Elizabeth: Do you look the same? Do you look like my good old brother Pete?

Pete: Hmm. I don't know, Sis. I haven't looked in a mirror, but I feel like me, just a lot better, like when I was younger.

Elizabeth: Do you have any trouble talking?

Pete: No, Sis, not at all. But it seems also I can just think things to people without speaking.

Elizabeth: Doesn't your mouth move at all? Do you have a mouth?

Pete: Not exactly. It's like a memory of a mouth or a thought of a mouth.

Elizabeth: Wow. It's hard to imagine.

Pete: It's hard to explain, Sis.

Elizabeth: Can you understand what others say to you?

Pete: Yes, of course.

Elizabeth: Well, that's good. What is the most amazing or surprising thing about where you are?

Pete: Oh, Sis, all the love. It is love all over.

Elizabeth: Sounds wonderful. Is there anything that you don't like?

Pete: Well, Sis, I miss you. I can't talk to you. Or rather, I have been trying to talk to you, but I guess you can't hear me.

Elizabeth: That's right. I have not heard you at all, but I can understand what you are saying now because somehow my arm hears you and writes your words. I'm getting sleepy, but I'll call you again tomorrow, okay?

Pete: We don't have tomorrow but call me when you can.

Elizabeth: Do you sleep?

Pete: I rest, but I don't need to sleep.

Elizabeth: Well, I have to say good night, Bro.

Pete: Good night, Sis. I love you, Sis. Thanks for being such a good sis. Sleep tight. Bed bug bite.

Elizabeth: Oh, Bro, bed bug bite.

SEPTEMBER 6, 2020

Elizabeth: I am eager to write. I especially hope I can talk with Pete. Pete, are you there?

Putty: Oh, dear woman, I want to rush to open the door for you, for your brother.

Elizabeth: Thanks, Putty.

Pete: Sis, I am here. I am here. And I am happy, so glad we can talk like this.

Elizabeth: So am I, Bro! I'm so excited. I like to think something wonderful could come of our talking—talking that might be good for others. Possible?

Pete: Sis, I am so new to this place where I am, but it is full of love, full of all possibility.

Elizabeth: I don't know if I could learn of another way of my hearing you. I am writing—that's how I listen and talk, but maybe I could learn another way, too.

Pete: Well, maybe, Sis. But we have this for now.

Elizabeth: Yes, Bro, can you see me right now as I write?

Pete: Yes, Sis, I can see you.

Elizabeth: Really?! You can see in the same way I see?

Pete: No, I don't think so. It's a different kind of seeing.

Elizabeth: Bro, you know this house where I live. You have been here many times. Do you remember it?

Pete: Yes, of course, Sis, and my room with my bed and TV.

Elizabeth: Yes, that's it. Can you see me in this house right now as we talk? Can you see where I am sitting?

Pete: Well, I know that you are sitting. I can feel your energy, your reaching to me.

Elizabeth: Can you see what I am wearing?

Pete: Is it flowers, Sis?

Elizabeth: Yes, Bro, I am wearing a bathrobe with flowers all over.

Pete: Sis, I don't think I am seeing it in the same way you're seeing it. I'm "reading" your seeing of it. It's different. If you think of something, whether you are seeing it or just thinking of it, I can sort of see your thinking. So, if you look at your bathrobe and think about what it looks like, I can see what you are thinking, but I don't really see you with my eyes or any eyes in the same way you are seeing with your eyes.

Elizabeth: Bro, you are explaining very well what is probably very hard to explain. But Bro, I get excited and happy when I think that I could learn a lot from you from where you are now.

Does that interest you at all—to tell me about where you are now?

Pete: If you want to do that, I can try to do that with you, Sis.

Elizabeth: Bro, I have so many questions. Is it okay to ask you? Would you tell me to stop if you don't want to do this?

Pete: Sis, you can ask me questions. If I can answer, I will try. Do you have a question now?

Elizabeth: Yes, Bro. This question is about you. Do you feel the same as when you were living, when you were alive on Earth all your sixty-three years?

Pete: Yes and no, Sis. I am sort of like who I was but also different. I am learning about this myself. I can recognize me as me, but I am also a bigger me, or a truer me—a me that includes the Pete you know but a lot more as well. I can think more clearly, move more easily—not so much struggle all the time. In my life I could not see well or hear well when I got older, but now a different kind of seeing and hearing is happening, and I like it. I like it very much.

Elizabeth: Oh, Bro, I am glad. I miss you. I am sad I cannot see you now, but I am so very glad that things are so good with you and we can talk like this. Would you be willing then to be a sort of teacher for me to help me understand your afterlife, the life you're living now after your life on Earth?

Pete: Sis, I will do what I can. I like the idea.

Elizabeth: Bro, can you tell me what you do when we're not talking? You don't have days and nights, right?

Pete: Not in the same way, Sis.

Elizabeth: So, what do you do?

Pete: Oh boy, this is a hard question because time isn't like time I knew before. I can do things, but not by time on the clock, so it's not always clear about when anything I do starts and finishes. No schedules, appointments, stuff like that.

Elizabeth: Bro, if you ever just want to tell me about anything at all—not just answers to my questions, please do. What I do is take some time—time, haha—every day or every few days, to sit quietly, maybe light a candle, and put myself into a trance, a sort of half-sleep, and then let my hand write. I'm doing that now. I'm sitting at my desk with a pad of paper and pencil. I say a little prayer and say I am ready to listen. Then I let my arm write on its own. That is how I am talking to you now and how I can hear what you're saying.

Pete: I guess maybe I knew that. That's good, Sis.

Elizabeth: Well, I'm about to stop now, but I'll do it again, call to you to see if you can talk, okay?

Pete: Yes, Sis. That's great. I like talking with you. Can we talk again soon? I love you, Sis.

Elizabeth: I love you too, Bro. Bed bug bite.

Pete: Bed bug bite, Sis.

SEPTEMBER 6, 2020

Elizabeth: Here I am, ready to write.

Pete: Hi, Sis! I am here. Can you hear me?

Elizabeth: Yes, I am writing your words and I can read your words that I write.

Pete: Oh, good. Sis?

Elizabeth: Yes, Bro?

Pete: How are you, Sis? Are you okay?

Elizabeth: Right now, I am fine, Bro. I am sitting in my bed and writing your words and mine. There are fireworks making a lot of noise near us outside. It's a holiday weekend and someone is shooting off the fireworks. I don't like the noise.

Pete: But we can talk anyway, can't we?

Elizabeth: Yes, Bro. Bro, I have a question.

Pete: What, Sis?

Elizabeth: What do you remember about the last part of your life?

Pete: Sis, I don't think I want to talk about that right now.

Elizabeth: Okay, Bro, maybe another time.

Pete: It was a sad time, and I don't like to think about it.

Elizabeth: Okay, Bro. Do you remember that we used to talk like this, you and I, through my writing? You would be sleeping, but you could talk in your sleep. I was in a sleepy-like trance, but I could write. Do you remember that? That wasn't sad, was it?

Pete: I remember that, Sis. I liked that, but it isn't so very clear in my thinking now.

Elizabeth: Well, at that time, you said you wanted to put our conversations into a book for others to read.

Pete: Yes, Sis.

Elizabeth: Do you remember that you said that?

Pete: I guess so, Sis.

Elizabeth: Well, Bro, it doesn't matter if you remember, but I can ask you now. Is it okay with you if I make these conversations you and I have into a book that others can read?

Pete: That's great. Will you do that, Sis?

Elizabeth: I will try to do it if it is okay with you.

Pete: Yes, of course, Sis, but do you think anyone would want to read it?

Elizabeth: I don't know. I hope so.

Pete: Well, Sis. Let's do it. We can talk, you write it down and make a book.

Elizabeth: If what we say is interesting, maybe some will want to read it.

Pete: I think so, Sis. Let's do it. Sis?

Elizabeth: Yes, Bro?

Pete: I left my life.

Elizabeth: Yes, you did. Now you're in the afterlife, right?

Pete: Yes.

Elizabeth: And have you been remembering and thinking about your whole life?

Pete: Yes, from when I was little.

Elizabeth: Can you remember all that?

Pete: Well, sort of. But others here are helping me to remember. I like some parts of my life. But other parts I don't like very much.

Elizabeth: Do you want to tell me about what you liked, what you didn't like?

Pete: I can say some. Some is happy, some is sad, some makes me angry. I like Mom and Dad, Mom especially because when I moved to live in New Jersey, she moved sort of close to me. She wasn't always easy, but I know she was always trying to help me. Dad tried to help too, but he was often busy working.

Elizabeth: Yes, true. Do you remember when we all lived on Clover Street in Rochester?

Pete: Yes, Sis, I remember. I remember my room, my blue chair, the little windows on one side and bigger windows on the other side. I liked that room. I didn't like going to school in New Jersey and then staying there. I was very sad then, but I tried not to show how sad I was.

Elizabeth: Oh, Bro. That must have been hard. I had moved out by then. But I remember visiting you in New Jersey.

Pete: I got used to it, Sis, but I was so so so very homesick.

Elizabeth: Oh, Bro, I'm so sorry. I know Mom and Dad wanted you to go to school, but there wasn't a school for you to go nearby.

Pete: But didn't they think how I would feel? I was so very young, and I knew no one at that school and where I lived there.

Elizabeth: Bye for now, more later.

Pete: Okay, Sis—bye for now.

This seems an abrupt ending. When writing while I was in trance, the trance itself could be shallow or deep. When deep, there was the risk that I might just fall asleep, which is what happened here. Sometimes when writing in trance, I was vaguely aware of what I was writing, even though I was not at all choosing my words, or Pete's, of course. But the depth of the trance did vary. Occasionally, when I came out of trance and read what I had written, I was surprised at what I found on the page because I had been deep enough not to be aware of the writing as I was writing. Luckily, most of the time, I was aware enough to be able to write legibly the words that showed up, but some were illegible.

SEPTEMBER 7, 2020

Elizabeth: I write and thank you all. I am lighting a candle. Pete, are you there?

Pete: Hi, Sis! I am here!

Elizabeth: Bro, it is morning here. I fell asleep last night when we were talking.

Pete: That's okay, Sis. How are you, Sis?

Elizabeth: I'm fine, Bro. I'm awake now, ready to talk. Will you tell me if you get tired or want to go do something else?

Pete: Yes, Sis, okay.

Elizabeth: Bro, are there things you want to tell me or ask me now?

Pete: Yes, Sis. I want to tell you that I wish we had more years in which we could have done more together as sister and brother. I had problems. You moved from the house. I moved to Bancroft. Mom was very much in my life, but you weren't until much later, especially when Mom died.

Elizabeth: Does it feel funny to say Mom "died?" Isn't she with you where you are? And aren't you both alive but living a different kind of life?

Pete: Yes, Sis. "Die" isn't the best word, but that's what people say. "Passed away" is better because it's like people just moved to a different kind of life. But the words are what people on Earth have created so they mean something to people living on Earth. I think many people don't know they can just move to a different kind of life.

Elizabeth: Bro, you sound so smart, so wise. Are you the same as when you were living on Earth?

Pete: No, Sis, I am different. Let's see if I can tell you. Well, for one thing, I can talk now. You know at the end of my life there I couldn't do that.

Elizabeth: Yes, I remember, Bro. I have to stop. I'll come back later.

Pete: Okay, Sis. That's okay. See you later.

Elizabeth: I open my heart and thank you all. Pete, Bigger Pete, are you there? I am ready.

Pete: Hi, Sis, I am here. It's Pete. How are you?

Elizabeth: I am fine, Bro. How are you? How is your life now?

Pete: Oh, Sis, if I had known here was so nice, I wouldn't have been so scared before I came.

Elizabeth: I'm glad. Anything you want to tell me or ask me now?

Pete: Sis, why didn't you come to see me at the new place I went to?

Elizabeth: Oh Bro, I arranged for you to move there for two reasons. First, you couldn't stay where you were living. You needed more nursing care than they could give you. The second reason was that I knew it was excellent, that they would take care of you well, and I could visit you more often because it is closer to our house.

But, when you moved in, there was a new disease in this country—COVID-19—which was very bad. The day after you moved in, they closed the doors where you were to visitors, and they would not allow me to visit you. It was for your safety and mine too, but I know it made us both sad. You probably remember we talked on the phone after that. Or rather, I talked, and you listened because you couldn't talk very well by then. You had lost language. But I called you when I couldn't visit. But then you got sick and sicker and that was it.

Pete: So, I died there.

Elizabeth: Yes, Bro, but remember how you just said that "die" is not a very good word because that life ended, it's true, but you have entered a new kind of life. And it sounds like a beautiful life.

Pete: Yes, Sis. I'm trying to understand the life I had and the life I'm having now.

Elizabeth: Bro, do you want to ask me anything about your life when you were here? I may be able to remind you of things. If you are taking time to think over your whole life, you can talk with me about it if you want to. My memory now is not so good, but I can tell you whatever I do remember. I can't say anything about where you are now. *You* are learning that. And I hope you will tell me about it. I want to know about where you are and how you are.

Pete: Why, Sis?

Elizabeth: Because I love you, Bro. I care about you and I hope you are okay.

Pete: Oh. And I'm glad you paid attention to me for so many years and helped me.

Elizabeth: Well, Bro, I did what I could, but I felt bad that I couldn't be with you at the end.

Pete: That wasn't your fault, Sis.

Elizabeth: You're right, Bro, but it felt like, still feels like, my fault and I'm sorry for that. Bro, you had a remarkable life. I learned a lot from you. I think, I hope, I can continue to learn from you.

Pete: What did you learn from me, Sis?

Elizabeth: One of the biggest things was that even though your body gave you difficulties, you complained very little, and you just kept going and finding things to smile and laugh about and enjoy.

Pete: I guess so. I'm glad for that but a lot of the time, I felt I just couldn't do things right or say things the right way.

Elizabeth: Yes, Bro. Some of that was because when you got older and your body didn't work so well, you became frustrated and angry. But then somehow you just got used to it. Or maybe you were angry inside but tried to be nice to those around you.

Pete: Yes, sometimes that happened.

Elizabeth: So, I was amazed that you could do that, that your body hurt or didn't work right, but you hardly ever complained.

Pete: Sis, that sounds pretty good.

Elizabeth: I'd say so, Bro. I learned to be more patient, to go with the flow, as they say.

Pete: Thanks, Sis.

Elizabeth: This is a long conversation. We can talk again, okay?

Pete: Okay, Sis, good idea.

Elizabeth: Okay, Bro, then I'll say goodbye now and send a hug.

Pete: Okay, Sis. Sis?

Elizabeth: Yes, Bro.

Pete: Take good care of yourself. I want you to have many more healthy years before you join me here.

Elizabeth: Thanks. One last question, Bro.

Pete: What, Sis?

Elizabeth: How often should we talk like this? I know you don't have days, nights, like here but do you have any suggestions now about how often we should talk or what we should talk about?

Pete: Not right now. But I'll think about it. Then I'll tell you.

Elizabeth: That sounds good, Bro. We can say goodbye for now.

Pete: Bye, Sis.

Elizabeth: Bye, Bro.

S E P T E M B E R   8 ,   2 0 2 0

Elizabeth: I am ready to write. I would be delighted to hear from any who wish to speak.

Mom: Hello, dear. I'm glad you and Pete are in contact.

Elizabeth: Yes, I am glad, too. I think you had something to do with that, yes?

Mom: Yes, dear, we were helping him to understand the special way you talk with those who have passed on.

Elizabeth: Thank you. I don't understand if it's Pete as I knew him or Pete's higher self or a combination, a merged soul who I am speaking with.

Mom: Well, dear, I don't know if I could explain it well because the lines are not so clear-cut, but you are observing well. Keep talking with him. I think it will become clear.

Elizabeth: Okay.

Mom: My sister is here, wants to say hello.

Aunt Elizabeth: Hello, Elizabeth. This is your Aunt Elizabeth. I have been wanting to speak with you.

Elizabeth: Really? About anything in particular?

Aunt Elizabeth: I wanted to be in touch. I think things are not easy now for you.

Elizabeth: True, many problems—Pete's passing and a worldwide disease that keeps us at home as vulnerable older people. There's horrible political division and climate change is much worse. Was there something specific you wanted to say?

Aunt Elizabeth: I wanted to cheer you on, to give you some support, encouragement—to let you know how many here are rooting for you.

Elizabeth: Well, that's good to know.

Aunt Elizabeth: And of course, I myself wanted to send love.

Elizabeth: Thanks, Aunt Elizabeth.

Aunt Elizabeth: You're welcome, my dear. Take good care of yourself. Times are hard. Do what you know helps you to sail through. You will.

Elizabeth: Well, that is definitely encouraging, thank you.

Aunt Elizabeth: Any time, my dear.

S E P T E M B E R 1 3 , 2 0 2 0

Elizabeth: I write. I open my heart and thank you all.

Pete: Hi, Sis.

Elizabeth: Hi, Bro. How are you?

Pete: I am fine, Sis. Everything is good. Now, do you have some of those questions?

Elizabeth: I want to ask you for any advice or suggestions about the book of these conversations. What is most important to say?

Pete: Okay, Sis. What is most important to say? It is important that people realize that there is so much more to life and death than we know, maybe much more than we can ever know. So that means it is important to keep learning and to keep humble and aware how little we know. And together that means we can share what we know with others and listen to them so we ourselves can learn. This is most important. We all have little pieces of the pie, a very sweet and nutritious pie, and we can share and feed each other.

Elizabeth: Nice, Bro. Very nice.

Pete: Also, Sis, everyone is capable of learning and sharing, even if it seems some might not be. So, the learning and sharing goes on. This is most important. Everyone is a learner; everyone is a teacher.

Elizabeth: Sounds good. That's fine, Bro. Goodbye for now.

Pete: Take good care of yourself, Sis.

Elizabeth: You too, Bro.

SEPTEMBER 15, 2020

Elizabeth: I write and thank you all. I am open to anything from anyone, Pete or others.

Mom: Hello, dear. I'm here with Pete. He wants to talk with you. He isn't sure he is doing this right.

Elizabeth: I have been able to hear from him as I put myself in a trance and let my arm write. This is the only way I know to communicate with you or him or anyone in the world of spirit, if that is the best phrase for where or how you exist.

Mom: You want to understand it, don't you?

Elizabeth: Yes, of course.

Mom: It's not preparation for your coming here now because I think it will be a long time before that happens. Pete?

Pete: Hi, Sis. Can you hear me?

Elizabeth: Yes, Bro. How are you? Nice to be with Mom, I guess.

Pete: Yes, Sis. Very nice and also nice to be with Dad and others.

Elizabeth: Are there those you didn't know before but are meeting for the first time there?

Pete: Yes, Sis, that's right. How did you know?

Elizabeth: I didn't know. That's why I was asking.

Pete: Oh. Sis?

Elizabeth: Yes, Bro?

Pete: You're writing a book, yes? About you and me and our conversations.

Elizabeth: Yes, we've talked about it, and you've given me some good ideas about it. Do you have some more thoughts?

Pete: I think it matters what the reason for the book is. I like to think it should be educational sort of. People can become more okay with life ending, then continuing.

Elizabeth: I think people would be interested to know what dying is like and what the afterlife is like. Maybe what it has been like for you is not like everyone, but it is one good and important story.

Pete: Yes, Sis, I am happy to tell what I can.

Elizabeth: Okay. Bro, do you think this is your story or my story?

Pete: Is that a question?! Sis, it's the story of both of us, brother and sister. Both of us.

Elizabeth: Yes, I think so.

Pete: Well, hmmm, what else, Sis? What is the name of the book?

Elizabeth: Right now, I am calling it *Bigger Pete.*

Pete: Why that?

Elizabeth: Because when we were talking before you passed on, there was your voice that somehow was able to talk with me while you were sleeping, but there was another voice which said he was your higher self. I called that voice Bigger Pete because he was you, my brother Pete, but a lot more too. He said he was all the lives you have lived. Do you know what I am talking about? Maybe you now are Pete, or maybe you now are Bigger Pete, that is my brother and a lot more too.

Pete: I can tell you this, Sis. I am not exactly the same as you knew me. I am different.

Elizabeth: Yes, I can tell. For one thing, you have no trouble talking now. And I think you have left all the troubles of your old physical body behind when you left this life.

Pete: Sis, I think you know a lot.

Elizabeth: Well, Bro, you told me a lot. You don't have a physical body now, do you?

Pete: No, Sis. But I am fine.

Elizabeth: Yes, you are probably much better now because your old physical body had lots of problems. You couldn't see well or hear well. You had Down syndrome, remember? You and I talked about that. That was your whole life long. Then at the end of your life you had a disease called Alzheimer's. Mom got that disease too before she passed away. That disease makes you forget things, even forgetting how to talk and understand language.

Pete: Sis?

Elizabeth: Yes, Bro?

Pete: The end of my life was hard.

Elizabeth: Yes, Bro, you had so many things that made your life hard, but what was amazing was how you hardly ever complained about it. Amazing.

Pete: Well, Sis, I couldn't talk well enough to complain, and I didn't understand what was happening to be able to tell it.

Elizabeth: Yes, Bro, that's because of the disease. It made all that so difficult. But I think all that was left behind when you passed on to where you are now. Right?

Pete: Right, Sis.

Elizabeth: So, I guess that feels really good not to have all those problems.

Pete: Yes, Sis, feels great. I feel fine. I feel I am the very best me, the truest me, the way I am supposed to be.

Elizabeth: That sounds wonderful, Bro. I am so glad, so very glad that I'd like to give you a big hug. But we can't do hugs now, can we?

Pete: Not those old hugs, no, but we can sort of feel the feel of hugs. It's love.

Elizabeth: Yes, Bro, true. Exactly. We can feel the feel of hugs which is love. Bro? You are sounding very wise, very smart. I like talking with you like this.

Pete: So do I, Sis, now that I know how to do it. I didn't know before, but Mom helped me. Dad helped me. Others too. I think you call them guides or angels or something.

Elizabeth: I'm glad you had the help. We'll talk again, but right now, my old hand is getting tired. Remember I have one of these old physical bodies that can get tired.

Pete: Oh, Sis, are you joking?

Elizabeth: Sort of, but it's true what I'm saying. I'll stop now, but talk with you again later, okay?

Pete: Okay, Sis. I love you, Sis.

Elizabeth: I love you too, Bro. Bye for now.

Pete: Bye, Sis.

CHAPTER NINE

PETE REVIEWS HIS LIFE

Elizabeth: I open my heart. Pete or Bigger Pete or other voices, I am ready.

Pete: Hi, Sis—it's me. I am fine, Sis. I like that we can talk this way again.

Elizabeth: Hi, Bro. So am I. Ready for questions?

Pete: I guess so, Sis. Go ahead.

Elizabeth: Bro, you said you were thinking about your life. Some call that a review of the life—life review. Is that it?

Pete: Yeah, Sis. I am thinking over my life—how it was, what I did, what I said, what was good, what not so good.

Elizabeth: Do you think about the purpose of that life?

Pete: Yes, Sis. That is a big and important piece.

Elizabeth: Do you think you chose that life somehow, that you chose our family to be born into, that you chose the challenges you would have?

Pete: Well, Sis, I am thinking about all that now and looking back over the whole life from start to finish. It takes a lot of thinking to sort things out.

Elizabeth: Have you learned anything new or is it too soon to know yet?

Pete: It's too soon, Sis. I'm working on it. Oh, I can tell you one big thing now. I am glad you are, or were, my sister.

Elizabeth: Am I still your sister?

Pete: Well, you were my sister in that life when I was Pete. Now I am still Pete and you are still Elizabeth, but I am different now. I am more than just Pete after his life as Pete. I've had other lives. I know that now. I am learning about all that.

But Sis, one thing is different here from that life where you still live. Earth life is physical, and things have clear material edges. Something is A, not B, or something is B, not A, and it's important to draw clear lines of difference between—what is called definition. But that is less important in a not-physical world. Or it's important but not in the same way.

Elizabeth: That is a clear explanation, Bro.

Pete: Sis, maybe that shows you I am not just Pete. Pete, your brother Pete, probably couldn't explain things like that very well, but I can now.

Elizabeth: Does that feel good to be able to do that now?

Pete: Yes, Sis. It's different from just Pete, and I sort of miss just Pete, but this feels like the real me, the true me, and that Pete, your brother Pete, was very frustrated not to be able to do things. I don't mean just at the end of that life but that whole life through. Pete, that Pete, wasn't very smart, couldn't think well or talk well or understand things. I'm remembering little by little how to do that now. And it feels like home, like the true home of me that I had forgotten in that life. I did what I could, but I couldn't do as much as I wanted.

Elizabeth: Wow, Bro. I am glad you are telling me this, but I am so sorry for the frustrations in that life. And I have to say, I think I never realized just how difficult things were for you. It seemed you were patient.

Pete: I tried, Sis—I tried.

Elizabeth: And you were so loving, so very loving.

Pete: That's all I had, Sis—all I had to offer, to give. I couldn't offer much else.

Elizabeth: Oh, Bro. If it's okay with you, I'm going to stop writing our conversation now, but I'll call again, and we can talk more. Okay?

Pete: Yes, Sis, of course. This is good for me. I hope it is for you.

Elizabeth: Yes and no, Bro. I'm sad and happy all at the same time. Big hugs, Bro. I'll call again.

Pete: Okay, Sis. Good, Sis. I love you, Sis.

Elizabeth: Here I am, ready to write for a while.

Pete: Hi, Sis—it's me. I am here. I can talk with you. I like this. Do you?

Elizabeth: Yes, Bro. Do you have anything to tell me or ask me?

Pete: Sis, why are you doing this?

Elizabeth: Bro, I miss you, so it's nice to talk. Also, I think together we can put together a collection of these conversations that others can read and learn about you, your life, your afterlife. I think many will learn from it, including me, Bro.

Pete: Oh, that's good. I do want to do it. Just asking. Sis, can you see me?

Elizabeth: Now?

Pete: Yes.

Elizabeth: No, I cannot see you or hear you, but the words in your thoughts seem to come to me and quickly go to my hand, which writes them. I can't hear them. I sort of think them in time to write them. Does that make sense? We were doing this when you were living, but always when you were asleep so your thoughts and words could travel on their own when your body was asleep on the bed. As for me, I was awake enough to write but in a sort of half-sleep, a trance, so I didn't control my questions to you but just wrote down what we somehow were able to say to each other.

Pete: That's cool, Sis. I didn't really know how it worked.

Elizabeth: I don't really know either. That's my best explanation. I don't think many people do it or do it as much as you and I have—maybe eight or ten years now, I'm guessing, or close to that.

Pete: Wow, Sis. The writing is cool—how we do it.

Elizabeth: Yes, you and me, Bro and Sis, together.

Pete: Nice. Now, your questions?

Elizabeth: Is Mom with you now?

Pete: No, but she's nearby. She helps me.

Elizabeth: That's good. Can you see her, and can she see you?

Pete: Not the way you're thinking of it, Sis. Everything is different. We rely on thoughts and feelings, not sight and sound. You can't see me, and I can't see you, so it's really amazing when you think about it that we can talk like this.

Elizabeth: True, Bro. I think it's hard to believe it, but we've been doing it a long time.

Pete: Yeah, Sis. Good for us!

Elizabeth: Bro, what do you do? Where do you go? What is the landscape where you are?

Pete: Oh boy, this will be hard to explain but I'll try. Sis, you know how you are always thinking?

Elizabeth: Yes.

Pete: Well, I still think here. I didn't realize how much thinking and feeling I did before because there was so much other stuff—body stuff, doing things with the body.

Elizabeth: Do you move?

Pete: Yes, Sis, I move, and very easily too, just by thinking myself in a direction. I'm getting used to it a little, but it's different. And it's so easy that I don't really notice how very different it is. I don't know if I can tell this well. But you'll see when you come. Not now, Sis, I know, but when you do. And Sis, when you come here, I want to show you around, help you get used to this place.

Elizabeth: Thanks, Bro. That's nice to know, but I don't want to come yet. I want to stay alive here for a number of years. So, I am being careful not to get sick. I have to stay at home almost all the time because of the virus that is a big disease all over the world now.

Pete: I'm glad you're careful, Sis.

Elizabeth: Bro, do you miss seeing and hearing things?

Pete: Oh, Sis, I'm not explaining well. I <u>can</u> see and I <u>can</u> hear, but not in the same way I did before or you do now. Because I was alive, I can think of something, and by thinking of it, I can see it, and I can hear it if it makes noise. But Sis, I can see things this way I don't think I could see when I was on Earth. It's sort of a soft seeing, not hard with edges. There is a lot to see, which is beautiful. And there is sound too which isn't noise but more like music, but that is softer too.

Elizabeth: Wow, Bro, hard for me to imagine.

Pete: Yes, Sis, I know.

Elizabeth: Bro, is there anything from living that you miss, that you wish for?

Pete: Yes, Sis. I miss some of my friends. I am sorry to have left them. And I miss you, but not quite so much when we talk like this.

Elizabeth: Is there stuff your body could do that you can't do now because you have no body?

Pete: Sis, first, that body of mine wasn't working too well. It was more frustrating than something I liked or enjoyed. And also, something else, Sis. I have a sort of body but it's different. It's me but it isn't skin and muscle and all that. It's different, hard to tell. It doesn't do the physical things my old body did or tried to do. It's way easier here.

Elizabeth: I am trying to understand. Can you sing or hum?

Pete: Oh, Sis, well, sort of, but again, not in the same way. Sis, I have an idea. Maybe somehow, I could come to you when *you* are asleep. Maybe I could somehow show you then. You know the way thoughts came to you into words when I was sleeping? Maybe I can send thoughts or picture thoughts to you when you are asleep so you can get an idea of what I am talking about.

Elizabeth: That would be wonderful, Bro, but I think I would forget when I wake up, just as you forgot our conversations when you got up before. I'm not really sure how it all works, but I am willing to try if you know when I am asleep. Oh, I could tell you when I'm going to bed, and maybe someone there could help you come in my thoughts like a dream. Then maybe you can show me, and I could learn what you are like and what it is like where you are.

Pete: Okay, Sis.

Elizabeth: Bro, this is a nice long talk, but I need to go cook dinner now, so we'll stop, okay?

Pete: Okay, Sis. Remember to tell me when you are going to sleep. It may take some time to learn how to do this, if it is even possible, but we can try.

Elizabeth: Yes, Bro. It will be a new learning for you and me. Goodbye for now.

Pete: Goodbye for now.

S E P T E M B E R   1 8 ,   2 0 2 0

Elizabeth: I am ready to write. I am open to Pete/Bigger Pete.

Pete: Hello, Sis.

Elizabeth: Hi, Bro. All well with you?

Pete: Yes, I am fine. You ask about Pete or Bigger Pete—who is talking? Pete's answer was good. Let me also explain. While the lines are not so clearly defined, as he said, I am the Bigger Pete part of Pete. The old Pete part of Pete has been talking with you, but try to understand that the old Pete is part of Bigger Pete. When you heard from me before, Pete was more separate because he was alive on Earth and I, Bigger Pete as you call me, have been Pete's higher self, not in a physical self.

Imagine it like this, like two overlapping circles. They were more separate before when Pete was alive, but now the circles of old Pete and Bigger Pete overlap much more. That isn't exactly the situation, but that picture may help you to understand.

Elizabeth: Yes, it does help, thank you.

Pete: It isn't easy to understand this world of spirit, but you have somewhere in your experience your own time here that you may have faint memories of. But a physical life on Earth does have a way of obliterating those memories so you can live properly on Earth. I hope this is clear.

Elizabeth: Yes, I would say very clear. Oh, I am getting sleepy.

Pete: Too early for that. You can sleep later. May we continue?

Elizabeth: Yes, yes, please! I think I can sort of tell the difference between the Bigger Pete and old Pete parts by the way you talk.

Pete: You realize we are not really talking.

Elizabeth: Yes, I understand that you don't have physical voices with the kind of sound that would be familiar to me.

Pete: That's correct. So, Pete's voice—old voice and Bigger Pete voice or voices—won't physically sound different.

Elizabeth: But your choice of words, the content of your words, seems to be expressed in a more formal way.

Pete: That's true. That's observant of you. And it is entirely appropriate as you have known your brother Pete—that is, old Pete—his whole life on Earth, but you and I have met only recently.

Elizabeth: True. So, I think I understand. It all makes sense.

Pete: Good. Now please feel free to ask me, Bigger Pete, anything, even if you have also asked Pete, old Pete. That way, you have his perspective and mine as well. He is learning about this world and doing beautifully so his fresh new seeing may serve to help explain things well. Now I think this is enough for this conversation.

Elizabeth: Okay.

SEPTEMBER 19, 2020

Elizabeth: I may get interrupted, but I want to try writing right away this morning. I am open to hear from anyone.

Mom: Hello, dear. Do your own work, <u>which is important</u>. Underline that and remember it. Pete is doing well. He is amazing. I am proud, if I can be, to have been his mother, to have born him and raised him.

Elizabeth: And you didn't shirk that even when others advised it.

Mom: True, my dear.

Elizabeth: And we all have gained from knowing him, and I continue to learn, to grow from knowing him. Are you near me now?

Mom: Yes, do you sense my presence?

Elizabeth: Sort of. I guess. Yesterday I felt quite a rush of presences near me as I wrote.

Mom: Yes, dear. First, you have much support from here—much. And you are becoming more aware, allowing yourself to become more aware of spirit presences. I know, we know you are skeptical, maybe a bit less so now. But your skepticism helps when it comes to sharing this work with others there who are skeptical. But your confidence and faith serve to bolster its acceptance by others. It makes you sound like more of an authority. And you have the authority of being the author of your writing so keep going, my dear daughter. That's all for now.

SEPTEMBER 21, 2020

Elizabeth: I sit to write. I open my heart, surrender my arm, and thank you all.

Pete: Hi, Sis, it's Pete and also the one you call Bigger Pete.

Elizabeth: Hello, Pete/Bigger Pete. I think I am understanding a little bit about the relationship between Pete/Bigger Pete. I wonder if these two overlapping circles of you will eventually merge entirely.

Pete: It's hard to say exactly.

Elizabeth: Can you say whether Pete's voice, as I know it, will eventually disappear?

Pete: We cannot say that either. There is much that Pete, as old Pete, is sorting out now about his life, and while not doing that entirely on his own, his voice to you can sound familiar.

Elizabeth: Oh, okay. I guess I am beginning to realize that Pete my brother, that is, old Pete, may disappear entirely later into Bigger Pete and I will lose him for a second time.

Pete: Oh, my, you're an observant one but also a worrying one. You need not worry because Bigger Pete, including old Pete, will be able to talk with you. And not only that, will be able to help you in so many ways in your life and understanding. This is Bigger Pete. Old Pete is involved with something now but will speak with you again later. Okay?

Elizabeth: Sure, fine.

SEPTEMBER 23, 2020

Elizabeth: I write and thank you all. I would be happy to hear from anyone.

Pete: Hi, Sis—it's Pete and Bigger Pete. I am learning about all this—what you call Bigger Pete. Things are changing here. I have to pay attention. It's not fast but things always seem to be changing. What are *you* doing?

Elizabeth: I'm sitting in my chair by my desk upstairs in my house. Do you remember the upstairs here? It has been a long time since you were able to climb stairs.

Pete: True, Sis. I bet I could now, except I have no legs. I would float up and down.

Elizabeth: Bro, can you visit my house, if you want to?

Pete: Yes, Sis, I think so, but why would I do that?

Elizabeth: I don't know. What people call ghosts are those in the spirit world that visit Earth. I don't know quite how it works. I don't know if we could see or hear each other if you came to visit.

Pete: I don't know either, Sis. I think others here would know, but not me. Or maybe I should say not yet. I am learning so much and, it seems, so quickly.

Elizabeth: How do you learn, Bro? Is someone teaching you?

Pete: Well, Sis—Mom and Dad help me. And then there are others I don't know from my old life who teach more like regular teachers or wise ones who tell you things. And then sometimes I just remember things I had forgotten.

Elizabeth: Why did you forget, Bro?

Pete: Sis, living my old life made me forget about this place. I had to pay attention to that life.

And, Sis, you know I wasn't so smart in that life.

Elizabeth: Well, Bro, but you were loving, and you taught me that being loving is better than being smart.

Pete: Oh, Sis—thanks, Sis. Well, guess what! Everyone here is so very loving. That's why it's so nice being here. You'll see. I know not now, but when you come.

Elizabeth: Sounds wonderful, Bro. Have you tried to visit when I am asleep? I have been telling you when I go to sleep.

Pete: Sis, I have been trying, but I don't know what I'm doing. When you did that as I was sleeping, you were writing, but it isn't like that

now. So, I'll keep trying or ask for help and maybe something will
work.

Elizabeth: Okay, Bro. It's okay whether it works somehow or not. Not
a problem at all, but I would certainly like to learn more about how
you are now and where you are now.

Pete: Sis, here's the important thing. I am fine where I am. I am happy
and free, and everything is good. So, I think that is most important,
yes?

Elizabeth: True, Bro, and knowing that, even though I can't see you now,
is a big relief. I am so glad you are fine—very glad.

Pete: Sis?

Elizabeth: Yes, Bro?

Pete: Keep things simple and let love in.

S E P T E M B E R 2 3 , 2 0 2 0

Elizabeth: Hello, all. I am here, ready to write the words of anyone or
groups or angels or guides—advice, guidance, whatever.

Unidentified voices: Hello, dear one on Earth. We will tell you not who
we are by name but ones who love you dearly, admire you, and wish
to support you. You have been in something of a lost time. You have
retired from teaching, retired from poetry, on your new stage of writing, your brother has gone, and you have this quiet, stay-at-home
retreat time, you're calling it.

Elizabeth: Yes, all true, all true.

Unidentified voices: We are here to say with all that going on, you are
doing beautifully, admirably well. Keep up all the good work. Now
we have some advice. Do <u>not</u> be tempted to get involved with political activism. That is not your role now. Stay with this work. Keep
your life simple and healthy. One of your biggest supporters is your
brother, who has returned home here. He is learning and remembering about everything here, and he is highly motivated to support you
in your work.

Elizabeth: Oh.

Unidentified voices: Yes, there is much for you ahead—new things, new learning, new surprises. So, carry on. You are leading a quiet life now. Keep it simple and some new things will gently open up and make themselves known to you.

Elizabeth: That's intriguing!

Unidentified voices: You are a dear one, well-loved, well-supported. It is perfectly okay and entirely appropriate in this time of your life to withdraw to do exactly what you are doing now.

Smile, dear daughter of Earth.

S E P T E M B E R   2 4 ,   2 0 2 0

Elizabeth: I write. I open my heart. I thank you all.

Pete: Hi, Sis. How are you, Sis?

Elizabeth: A bit tired of having to stay home all the time because of the disease outside.

Pete: Disease, Sis?

Elizabeth: Yes, it's a virus called COVID-19. I think that may be what caused the end of your life.

Pete: How do you know that, Sis?

Elizabeth: I am not certain, but you had a high fever, and medicine didn't help to bring it down. Also, you had trouble breathing. Remember the oxygen mask you had to wear?

Pete: Yes, Sis.

Elizabeth: I think that was the disease.

> *It was quite possible that Pete had COVID-19. There were cases of it, both staff and residents, at the nursing home. Pete, who was in a vulnerable state anyway, developed the symptoms of unrelenting high fever, lack of oxygen, and extreme fatigue. But this was early on in the pandemic, and he was not tested for the virus. The death certificate did not indicate COVID-19 as cause of death.*

Bro, you were not very well then. That's why I arranged for you to move to the nursing home. They couldn't take good care of you where you were. Also, I wanted to be able to visit you more, and the nursing home was much closer.

Pete: Oh, okay, Sis. I am not sorry to be done with that life. It was getting very hard.

Elizabeth: Yes, Bro. You were very patient while your body had lots of troubles.

Pete: Sis, I am fine here.

Elizabeth: That's good. I am glad. Bro?

Pete: Yes, Sis?

Elizabeth: Do you know what I mean if I say you have a higher self there where you are?

Pete: Sis, I am learning many new things. Sometimes I know that I am not just the brother you know but more besides.

Elizabeth: Yes, Bro, I think that is what I am talking about—a higher self, a bigger Pete that you are part of but is a whole lot more.

Pete: Well, Sis, I do feel smarter than I did in my life. It is easier for me to learn and remember new things, and I like that. I like it very much. But, Sis, it is different and strange. It's almost as if I don't always recognize my own self, but who I am here, who I am remembering as me, is also somehow familiar. It's strange but it feels good, right, not scary or wrong. It just takes some getting used to.

Elizabeth: You are telling it well, Bro.

Pete: Sis?

Elizabeth: Yes, Bro?

Pete: I think this is all I can say now, but let's talk again. Take good care of yourself. Live a good life. Come later, much later, and until then, or at least for now, we can talk.

Elizabeth: Sounds good to me, Bro.

Pete: Okay then, bye. Oh, remember bed bug bite?

Elizabeth: Right, Bro—bed bug bite.

Elizabeth: Here I am ready to write. I would be happy to hear from whoever wishes to speak.

Pete: Hi, Sis.

Elizabeth: Hi, Bro. How is everything going?

Pete: Mostly wonderful.

Elizabeth: Mostly only?

Pete: Well, there is a lot going on, and well, it's mostly wonderful. Sis?

Elizabeth: Yes, Bro?

Pete: I'm thinking about my life. Do you remember when I was born?

Elizabeth: Yes, some.

Pete: What can you tell me?

Elizabeth: I remember how big Mom's stomach was before you were born, and I remember when you were born that Mom and Dad found out you had Down syndrome and that would make some things in life difficult for you. Bro, is there a reason, or did you have any choice about being born with Down syndrome?

Pete: Sis, that's one thing I am learning and remembering now about choosing what I did about that life. I'll tell you later, but I myself am right in the midst of figuring that out.

Elizabeth: Oh, Bro, you are amazing. Please tell me anything you want to share or ask me any questions.

Pete: I just did. Any other memories?

Elizabeth: Yes, Mom thought you should have a strong name to help you with any difficulties you might face.

Pete: So, Pete is a strong name?

Elizabeth: From the Bible. Well, Peter—you shortened it to Pete.

Pete: Oh, okay.

Elizabeth: Why did you shorten it to Pete? Because of that sports guy?

Pete: Sis, to me, Pete sounded better, stronger, manly.

Elizabeth: Oh. Once you decided on Pete, you didn't like it all when people called you Peter, mostly people that didn't know you well didn't know you really liked Pete much better. If I was somewhere with you, I'd clue them in.

Pete: Oh, Sis. I guess maybe I know that. Thanks.

Elizabeth: You're welcome, Bro.

Pete: You're cool, Sis.

Elizabeth: Oh well, thanks, Bro—you're pretty cool, too.

SEPTEMBER 28, 2020

Elizabeth: I write, surrender my arm, open my heart, and thank you all.

Dad: I am here—your father.

Elizabeth: Oh, Dad, I dreamt of you dressed in gray with white shirt and tie. I was so glad to see you, but I woke up too quickly.

Dad: I show my support in what ways I can. Pete has been saying such wonderful things of you, how you helped him in his life and now still try to stay in touch with him. I am here to say what a marvelous sister you have been to him, and I thank you. I could have been a better father, but I am doing what I can now.

Elizabeth: Dad, it's wonderful to hear from you. You were a good father. We do what we can when we can, yes?

Dad: Ah, you see? That's your loving spirit showing.

Elizabeth: Pete has been my example. It took me a long time to see it, but he is a being of love. I don't know how he managed so well, but, well, he's there with you all now and he says he's fine.

Dad: He is. And he is welcome and well-loved. I am proud to be, or to have been, his father in that life.

Elizabeth: It's good to hear you say that.

Dad: And I'll be glad to see you when you come here—but not now!

Elizabeth: Okay.

Dad: Call me again anytime.

OCTOBER 6, 2020

Elizabeth: I am ready to hear from anyone. I open my heart to write your words.

Pete: Hi, Sis!

Elizabeth: Hi, Bro. How are you doing? Are you learning things?

Pete: Yes, Sis. That's mostly what I do. It takes up most of the time, but there really isn't time here.

Elizabeth: How do you manage?

Pete: It's different from how you're probably thinking. I think it's easier to come together with others. No clocks, letters, travel. Thinking is how people come together.

Elizabeth: Do you sleep?

Pete: No, but sometimes I am quiet or resting but not because I am tired. I don't really get physically tired because there's not much physical here. What I've been learning is how things work but also thinking about my life and what I learned from that. It was so different from other lives because I was so dependent on the help of others.

> *I was curious about Pete's mentioning other lives. I wondered whether he meant the lives of other people or maybe other lives he had lived. But when in the trance state, I did not have conscious control over what I said or asked. So, in spite of my curiosity, that question did not get asked.*

Elizabeth: Oh, Bro, I had a dream about that, about my wanting to be independent, and for some reason, that you wanted a life where you depended on others.

Pete: Yes, Sis—that's it.

Elizabeth: You didn't even bother with money, and it's hard to have a life here these days without paying at least some attention to money.

Pete: I needed to do the basic things of eating, sleeping, and so forth, but not so much else, especially at the end of that life. When I was in school and working, I had to do things, but mostly I did what people showed me to do. Sometimes it was very frustrating that I couldn't do as much as others or think as well as others, especially when it got harder and harder even to talk. Sis?

Elizabeth: Yes, Bro?

Pete: What did you think of my life?

Elizabeth: Oh my, what can I say? Well, let me start with how loving you were. That was true all the way through. I don't remember your being mean or nasty. If things weren't going well, you would just back away or refuse to participate. And you were very patient with all the difficulties you faced.

Pete: Not always, Sis.

Elizabeth: Well, it seemed so.

Pete: Thanks. Sis?

Elizabeth: Yes, Bro?

Pete: Sis, be careful. Stay healthy. Don't get sick.

Elizabeth: Okay, Bro, thanks. That's what I am trying to do. We'll talk later.

Pete: Okay, Sis. I love you. Let's talk again.

O C T O B E R 7 , 2 0 2 0

Elizabeth: I open my heart, surrender my arm, and thank you all.

Putty: Hello, dear little spark of life on Earth.

Elizabeth: I'm never clear whose thoughts are whose these days. It doesn't help to have an old brain.

Putty: Your brain is fine. Keep going. Keep writing, dear little spark. I'll open the door.

Pete: Hi, Sis! It's me—Pete—and Sis, I'm not exactly as you knew me, just as Pete, your brother.

Elizabeth: Can you tell me how you are different?

Pete: I'll try, Sis. I knew you would ask, Question Lady!

Elizabeth: Are you more or less or just different?

Pete: More _and_ less _and_ different. I am less of the Pete with Down Syndrome and Alzheimer's disease. Those were of my body. And I have less of that body. I am more healthy, more smart, more able to move, to learn, to think, to remember. My mind is active and eager and remembering I am more than just Pete, more than that life. I <u>have</u> lived before. I am learning about that.

Elizabeth: Have you learned of lives that you and I shared? Where we knew each other?

Pete: Oh yes, Sis. Quite a few. Do you mind if I call you Sis?

Elizabeth: Why should that bother me?

Pete: Well, I have been changing, and I'm out of the life where I was your brother.

Elizabeth: But that's how I know you best, or rather the part of you I know best.

Pete: But Sis, we may discover other lives where we have known each other, and maybe Sis wouldn't work in those lives.

Elizabeth: Okay. True. I'm still me, may be changing a little now but not so dramatically as you.

How shall we call each other? Any suggestions?

Pete: How about Pete Plus?

Elizabeth: Sure, I can call you Pete Plus.

Pete: I have learned about higher selves. We all have souls—the core of who we are—and not all of that soul comes into life on Earth when one is born into an incarnation. Some people call the whole thing—life on Earth or lives on Earth plus the part of the soul that remains in the world of spirit—that whole thing is often called the higher self.

Elizabeth: Your higher self has spoken to me through this writing. It sounds more like you now—yourself but with more. I was calling that higher self Bigger Pete, which sounds to me what you might call Pete Plus. I'm not sure if the name is important, but it helps to understand what's going on and who one is speaking with.

Pete: Oh, okay.

Elizabeth: What would you like to call me now, then?

Pete: Hmm, I'll have to think about it. Old Sis? Old Elizabeth? I don't know. Oooo—how about Soulmate Sis?

Elizabeth: That sounds strange coming from you. Soulmate? I don't know. Maybe we can both think about the names and, meanwhile, just use Bro and Sis until some other names come to our thinking that might be better.

Pete: Okay. Sis?

Elizabeth: Yes, Bro?

Pete: Do you want to hear more about me now?

Elizabeth: Yes! Yes!

Pete: Well, you already know I don't have a body. That is, not the body I had as Pete. But, Sis, I have another, a different kind of body, more like a bunch of energy. It's like my mind but with more powers to it. That is, I can do more things, make things happen. Sort of like superheroes or magic. Maybe any mind in an Earth body could do such things, but mine certainly could not. Without the distraction and demands of my physical body, my mind feels stronger, seems stronger. Does this make sense?

Elizabeth: Sort of.

Pete: And something else, Sis. What the physical body, any physical body, does is keep its identity with certain edges or borders. Each body has a clear physical boundary where it stops. But minds don't have boundaries like that. It is more fluid. I am mostly my own mind, but where does my own mind stop and some other mind begin? Even in a physical Earth body, you just cannot answer that. But the brain? The brain is physical and has definite edges to its parts—lobes, cells, synapses—all that stuff.

Elizabeth: Wow, Bro, you *are* learning a lot!

Pete: Well, yes, but you see, even now as I talk with you, my own mind can borrow ideas, can borrow things to tell you, sort of like what people write and then footnote to say it was someone else's idea. That's very important when bodies have definite boundaries and bodies have names to identify them and what belongs to one body is so important. But you see, here there is not all that. Minds can share ideas, and no one insists on claiming an idea as their own alone. Does this make sense?

Elizabeth: It's beautiful, Bro. Yes, it makes sense.

Pete: Well, so you see, if you call me Bro the way you did when I was just Pete, that makes sense, but now I am that Pete still, sort of, but so much more. It's not that I, by myself, am so smart but that, as I talk, I can borrow thoughts to help say what I am saying. People here help each other. People cooperate. They don't just hold onto their own thoughts and not share. There is sharing and loving and helping, not fighting and hoarding.

Elizabeth: Sounds nice, Bro.

Pete: Do you understand?

Elizabeth: I think so. And I'm so glad you are telling me.

Pete: See, Sis—selfish doesn't work here. Of course, when people first come, if they are selfish, it's a big change, but most see it, as far as I know, as a good change. And Sis, I think you get it because you are not a selfish person.

Elizabeth: Oh, thanks, but I think I can be as selfish or more selfish than other people.

Pete: I don't see it.

Elizabeth: Well, thanks. If I am loving and sharing and unselfish at all, I think I have learned a good bit of that from you. When you were living as Pete, you were not selfish but loving and giving.

Pete: Aw, shucks, Sis, thanks.

Elizabeth: Well, Bro, I'm going to stop this writing, this conversation now, but let's talk again.

Pete: Sure, Sis. Sis, for now. Anytime. I love you, Sis. Take good care of your wonderful self (what you always said to me).

Elizabeth: Okay. Bye, Bro.

O C T O B E R   8 ,   2 0 2 0

Elizabeth: I open my heart, surrender my arm, breathe in the cosmos, and thank you all, including Pete, Bigger Pete, or anyone else.

Pete: Hi, Sis.

Elizabeth: Still using Sis? Did you think about better names?

Pete: Oh, Sis—I guess Sis and Bro are okay. It's how we know each other, at least in my most recent life, the one you are still in.

Elizabeth: Bro, okay. I did a past life session with a man in England. I discovered we shared a life long ago where we were both in a religious order. You were older than me, a protector of me. I would do lots of writing of voices I heard but from people or such I couldn't see. I don't know if I was very smart in that life. I never married but stayed in the religious order where you were. You were so very kind, so loving—like now.

Pete: Oh, Sis, I'm glad I was kind.

Elizabeth: Bro, if you learn anything about that life or others we've shared, let me know, will you?

Pete: Okay. Sis?

Elizabeth: Yes, Bro?

Pete: Are you okay?

Elizabeth: Well, not at my best. The disease—COVID-19—still means we have to stay at home, cannot go out, and of course I miss you too, so I'm not at my best. And our country is not at its best either. I don't know if you know what is going on but many problems. An election is coming up soon.

Pete: Sis, I've been paying attention mostly to what I'm doing here, but yes, I know things are not good. I hope you and everybody can stay safe and well and kind.

Elizabeth: Thanks, Bro. I hope so too. Bro, I have lit a candle here. Can you see it?

Pete: Not the same way you can. But once you look at it and tell me, then yes, I can sort of, but not with eyes but by being with you in our minds.

Elizabeth: Can you say more?

Pete: Sis, you are the writer, not me.

Elizabeth: But Bro, this is about where you are now, not about where I am.

Pete: Well, true, Sis. It's a way of talking and seeing through our minds, not with mouths or eyes.

Elizabeth: That makes sense. Bro?

Pete: Yes, Sis?

Elizabeth: Do you feel any pain at all?

Pete: It's sort of the same. I don't have physical pain. I don't have a physical body, but I do feel a different kind of aching or longing for things on Earth to be better. Those here try to help Earth in what ways they can. I want to learn how to do these things so I can help those on Earth, not just all the people (including you, Sis) but all the animals, birds, fish, who are having a hard time now.

Elizabeth: Are you talking about changes in the climate?

Pete: Yes, that, but so many things. Human beings are supposed to have free will to make decisions, but first, there are so many human beings now, and so many do not make good decisions.

Elizabeth: How can you or anyone where you are help with that?

Pete: Well, for one thing, Sis, those on Earth must want the help. Not all do. Some know how to pray, and they do. Some ask for help in other ways, but there are just so many that are suffering and don't know how or don't have the energy or resources to help themselves.

Elizabeth: Wow, Bro, you are sounding so wise, as loving and caring as ever, but you are talking about things that you didn't talk about in your life. I am glad. I am impressed and just a bit sad we didn't have these conversations when you were here.

Pete: But we're talking now, Sis, and it's good, very good. You are kind and loving and concerned. You are doing what you can.

Elizabeth: Perhaps I could do more. I wonder how I could do more help without going out and getting sick.

Pete: Sis, you are best doing what you are doing. Someone has to stay quiet and sane and thoughtful and help others from a distance. I hope you can take care of yourself and stay well. A time will come when you can go out more safely. You need not feel bad to stay quiet at home.

Do it. You're doing fine. As you always said to me, take good care of your wonderful self.

Elizabeth: Thanks, Bro. In fact, talking with you like this helps me to feel better.

Pete: Then, Sis, maybe our words will help others.

Elizabeth: Well, Bro, as you know, I am typing up all our conversations and plan to make the book as we spoke of before.

Pete: And that you <u>promised</u> to do, Sis.
Elizabeth: Yes, Bro.
Pete: Okay, then, let's stop now, but we'll talk again.
Elizabeth: Okay. Bye for now, Bro.
Pete: Bye for now, Sis.

O C T O B E R 11, 2 0 2 0

Elizabeth: Here I am, ready to write. I wonder if any might suggest how I might use this connection better between myself and all of you in spirit.

Putty: Hello, dear Elizabeth—this is your Putty, your Theodore, your Ted, your Teddy.
Elizabeth: Oh my, all that now?!
Putty: I like the idea of your calling me Teddy. It sounds so cozy.
Elizabeth: I can call you that if you prefer.
Putty: Try it.
Elizabeth: Okay.

I said okay to calling Putty "Teddy," but I was too many years in the habit of referring to him as Putty in these conversations to change now. To call him Putty was his own request when he first appeared because he was, when alive, a famous American poet, and he thought it might be distracting for me to call him by his name as a famous poet. Maybe his mentioning his name at this point indicated that he thought that using his real name might no longer be an issue.

Putty: I'll open the door.
Elizabeth: Thank you.
Unidentified voices: Hello, Elizabeth, dear daughter of Earth. There are those of us who wish to guide you to finish this part of your writing—what will be the book about your brother. This is your work now. Minimize your other work. You will have more inside time now. You will have all the help you need. This will not be your last book, but you cannot get to the next one before you finish this, so make your schedule and get going. That's all.

OCTOBER 14, 2020

Elizabeth: I am ready. I light my candle.

Pete: Hi, Sis. How are you?

Elizabeth: I am okay, Bro. How are you?

Pete: I am happy, free, and sort of excited.

Elizabeth: Why are you excited, Bro?

Pete: I am learning about so many things.

Elizabeth: Like what? Can you tell me?

Pete: I am learning how to think about my life as Pete. There are things I could have done better, but it was a brave life, and I did it rather well.

Elizabeth: That's great, Bro. It wasn't an easy life because, physically, you had difficulties. Can we talk about Down syndrome now? And the last years were hard with Alzheimer's. Have you talked to Mom about that? She had that disease too. So, you had hardships. The easier part was that Mom did her best to provide for you, to make sure you had the help you needed. It may have been lonely for you when you went so young away to school, but she wanted you to have the best help, and there was nothing closer to our house.

The most amazing thing was your own patience through all your years. What I do not understand was whether your soul or your higher self actually chose such a hard life and, if so, why.

Pete: Oh, Sis, you have thought about my life. I wish we could have talked more about it when I was living.

Elizabeth: Bro, don't you remember? You did not want to talk about it. You didn't want to admit it or to focus on any disability. That, it seems to me, was your own choice.

Pete: Yes, that's true. I thought that was a smart choice, that I could just ignore the fact of any disability. I wasn't thinking well, I suppose, but people with Down syndrome don't always think too well. But, Sis, I think in some ways it was a good choice because I couldn't be angry or think of myself as a victim if I didn't even acknowledge there was a problem.

What *really* made me angry was when I got Alzheimer's disease. It just seemed like one huge burden on top of the rest. I was very angry.

You told me some of it was about getting older. What you also told me, the most important part that I held like a treasure, was you said you would help me with whatever I needed, that you were still my sister and ready to do what would make my life better, that I wouldn't have to do it alone. Sis, that was your big gift to me—that you would stand by me.

Elizabeth: Yes, Bro, I said that, and I meant it and tried my best to do it. Thank you for telling me how much it meant to you. I remember I was at a conference in Florida when your doctor told me about the Alzheimer's disease. It made me so upset, so very upset, because I saw what the disease was like for Mom. I thought it so unfair, so difficult, and I didn't know what it would be like for you. I cried and cried. And then I thought about how to talk with you about it. And then I decided that I would not travel far but be close enough to come to you if things got rough.

And they did—not just Alzheimer's, but the falls, the accidents, the hospital trips—everything. Bro, you went through a lot. The mystery to me is whether or not we actually choose to have such lives, to be born with built-in difficulties. I don't know the answer to that one.

Pete: I'm not sure I know either, Sis, but that's a part of what I am learning. The thing is, it may not be choosing all the details of a life but some aspects of it that then play out as one goes through. The issue of dependence was a big one. To have to rely on the help of others is a big issue.

That's why your saying to me you would help was so important. The first time you said it was in the car. You were driving. We were between my place and yours. You reassured me that when difficulties came, you would be there to help me. You said it as if it was no big deal. That itself softened the whole thing about dependence. That if I became even more dependent, you would just easily be there for me. So, it made the dependence less terrible. Do you understand?

Elizabeth: Wow, Bro, yes, I think I do. I remember that conversation. I told you some of the things that might become difficult, like not remembering things, not being able to do things, not being able to say what you wanted to say. I knew some of that because that's what happened with Mom when she got Alzheimer's.

Pete: That's right, Sis. She had that experience, and she didn't have Down syndrome, so, well, I don't have it now. I can think clearly and review my whole life. I can remember my life, and Sis, you were such a big part of it, especially after Mom died.

Elizabeth: Yes, Bro, but maybe not such a big part before that. Mom really looked out for you. She never stopped, even though she got Alzheimer's. She couldn't do much at that point.

Pete: Sis?

Elizabeth: Yes, Bro?

Pete: Sis, with all the difficulties, it's good when people can keep each other company and help when necessary.

Elizabeth: True, Bro. Very true. There is a saying I heard once, supposedly from Vietnam, that hell was where the chopsticks were so very long that one couldn't even feed oneself, but in heaven, even though the chopsticks were just as long, people fed each other. Beautiful, yes?

Pete: That's nice, Sis. That's it. Sis, I am glad we were sister and brother.

Elizabeth: So am I, Bro. So am I.

Pete: Sis, I want to help you now as you tell our story.

Elizabeth: I'm glad, Bro.

Pete: Take good care of yourself. Work hard but not too hard. Take good care of your wonderful self.

Elizabeth: Thanks, Bro. Bye for now.

OCTOBER 19, 2020

Elizabeth: I am ready to write. My question is: Am I done with collecting conversations with you, Pete and Bigger Pete, and is it time to pull it into a book?

Unidentified voices: We come to you, the voices without names. Yes, it's good now to complete this work. We would say congratulations but not quite yet. Continue the final touches.

Elizabeth: Thank you. I'm so glad for your response.

Unidentified voices: You are welcome. Also, the communication lines are still open. You do not need to close that off. You will find other treasures in this way. Aren't you curious?

Elizabeth: Oh, yes. Yes!

Unidentified voices Well, then, get on with your work.

210 · BIGGER PETE

Pete: I'm still here. I'm not saying goodbye at all. I only say the book
project is ending. Call me anytime.

Elizabeth: Okay, I——

Peter: I love you, Sis. Bye for now.

N O V E M B E R   2 ,   2 0 2 0

Elizabeth: Here I am, I rest in the procection and wisdom of Divine
Light and Love.

Peter:

Elizabeth: Hi, Bro—always nice to hear from you. How are you?

Pete: Oh Sis, I am so happy to be here. I am doing many
things. I am looking over my whole life. Some parts I don't want to
see.

Elizabeth: That——

Peter: But Sis, I think I did——

Elizabeth: Yes, Bro.

Peter: Sis,

Elizabeth: Yes, Bro?

Peter: Sis,

Elizabeth: Yes, Bro?

Peter: Sis,

Elizabeth: Yes, Bro?

so there willing to be, and stories to be written now.
People should be told.

Elizabeth: I agree, Bro. I hope and pray for the same.

Peter: Thank them in front of me now, but as they, again, see and loved
you about what I am doing and learning.

Elizabeth: Okay, Bro.

— CHAPTER TEN —

PETE AND BIGGER PETE
COME TOGETHER

O C T O B E R   2 1 ,   2 0 2 0

Elizabeth: I am ready to write. I would be happy to hear from Pete Bigger Pete.

— ⌇ —

Pete: Hi, Sis—it's Pete and Bigger Pete. Sounds like you are ready to finish the book.

Elizabeth: Yes, I am. Any suggestions for it?

Pete: Well, yes. First, keep doing what you are doing. You may need to add some contextual material but as little as possible. Keep at it. Don't stop. That's most important. Sis?

Elizabeth: Yes?

Pete: I am so glad you have been doing this. I am beginning to understand it better now as I am beginning to understand so many things better. I would like to continue the conversations with you, but I think it is good to stop and put the book together now. It needs to be finished, be published, be read. Sis?

Elizabeth: Yes?

Pete: I have said it many times, but I say it again. Thank you—a big thank you.

Elizabeth: I hear you, Bro, and I thank you as well. I think you are busy now with your afterlife.

Pete: Yes. And Sis?

Elizabeth: Yes, Bro?

Pete: I'm still here. I'm not saying goodbye at all. I only say the book project is ending. Call me anytime.

Elizabeth: Okay, Bro.

Pete: I love you, Sis. Bye for now.

N O V E M B E R   3 ,   2 0 2 0

Elizabeth: Here I am. I trust in the protection and wisdom of Divine Light and Love.

Pete: Hi, Sis.

Elizabeth: Hi, Bro—always nice to hear from you. How are you?

Pete: Oh, Sis. I couldn't be happier. I am so happy. I am doing many things. I am looking over my whole life. Some parts I don't like to see.

Elizabeth: Bro, that's probably true for everyone. It certainly would be for me.

Pete: But Sis, I think I did it okay.

Elizabeth: Bro, you were splendid. You have always been so loving toward others and so patient with all the troubles you had.

Pete: Sis?

Elizabeth: Yes, Bro?

Pete: I am rather busy, but I know there was an election.

Pete had always been interested in politics and voted conscientiously in every election until he declined with Alzheimer's.

No more voting for me, but I hope all is well and that turmoil is low. People should be kind.

Elizabeth: I agree, Bro. I hope and pray for the same.

Pete: That's all from me for now. But do call me again, Sis, and I'll tell you about what I am doing and learning.

Elizabeth: Okay, Bro.

NOVEMBER 16, 2020

Elizabeth: Here I am, ready to write. Pete, are you there? If you're busy, I can try again later.

—☺

Pete: Hi, Sis!

Elizabeth: Hi, Bro. How are you?

Pete: Sis, I am fine and happy. I am very near you right now. Do you know that?

Elizabeth: No, I didn't. Can you see me?

Pete: Not the way you're thinking. But I feel that you are sitting down.

Elizabeth: Yes, I am, and I am writing with my pencil on my yellow pad of paper. Can you see what I am wearing?

Pete: Sis, I don't know if I can tell exactly. A big sweater? Sort of pebbly looking gray?

Elizabeth: Yes, Bro—a big black, gray, white knit sweater—bulky big knitting.

Pete: Sis?

Elizabeth: Yes, Bro?

Pete: I can "see" better here because it doesn't need eyes, physical eyes.

Elizabeth: I wish I could understand better.

Pete: You'll see when you come here.

Elizabeth: Have you been coming into my dreams?

Pete: Yes, Sis.

Elizabeth: But I can't remember when I wake up. So, I am taking a dream class. I think the teacher will tell how to remember dreams better.

Pete: That's good. Sis, call me again. I like talking with you.

NOVEMBER 16, 2020

Elizabeth: I sit to write. I ask for Pete or Bigger Pete but am happy to hear from anyone.

—☺

Pete: Hi, Sis—this is Pete and Bigger Pete together.

Elizabeth: Hello, Bro and Bigger Pete. Are you one or two people?

Pete: Oh wow. We probably should explain. But it's not easy. We're actually one *and* two. We are really one and the same. Pete is a part of Bigger Pete, but Pete separated into a life on Earth as your brother. That'll probably have to do for now.

Elizabeth: Okay, Pete. I miss you.

Pete: Sis?

Elizabeth: Yes, Bro?

Pete: Do not miss me. I mean, do not feel sad I am gone from that life. It was hard, especially at the end. Where I am now is much better. You should feel happy when you think of me now.

Elizabeth: Okay, Bro. I hear you. You didn't have an easy life, but you made it into a good life.

Pete: Sis, we can talk at another time. Bed bug bite.

Elizabeth: Yes, Bro, bed bug bite.

NOVEMBER 17, 2020

Elizabeth: I open my heart and thank you all.

Putty: Hello, dear, loyal, dedicated one. You are ready to hear whatever comes. I open the door.

Elizabeth: Thank you, Putty. Is the veil so thin between you and me, between my world here and the world of spirit?

Putty: Yes, my dear, very thin—indeed so thin you cannot believe it, cannot believe you can cross it so easily. Yes, you can. You're doing it, dear one. Don't doubt. Trust. Listen.

Elizabeth: Thanks, Putty.

NOVEMBER 18, 2020

Elizabeth: I sit to write and wonder who would like to speak.

Pete: Sis—hello, Sis.

Elizabeth: Hi, Bro. How are you?

Pete: I am learning a lot, and I like to be learning about my life and also how this life—this afterlife/between lives—works.

Elizabeth: Bro, what are you learning about your life as Pete? Did you choose that life?

Pete: Yes, Sis, in a way, I did. Not all the details, but I wondered what it would be like to be so dependent on others. I had had other lives where I was very independent and lives where I helped others who were dependent on me. I didn't always like those dependent people. They seemed lazy, and it wasn't always clear that they truly needed help or even wanted it. I was impatient with them. I couldn't imagine what it would be like to need so much help. Well, as Pete, I found out, especially at the end. Didn't you get impatient with me, Sis, when I was so dependent, when I needed so much help?

Elizabeth: No, Bro, not really, because you didn't live with me. People at Bancroft helped you most of the time. When you came here, I knew that you could not do some things. It wasn't laziness. It was what people call a disability.

One time I was upset because you had been given some medicine that made you even more unable to do things, so I was upset with the doctor but not with you. I was upset with you when you got in your stubborn moods, like when you wouldn't get in the car for me to drive you back. I realize now that saying no as you did was a way of your being strong, but it sure wasn't easy. Also, you didn't want to take baths or showers, but you wouldn't let me bathe you. So, I didn't like that. But Bro, most of the time you were a delight to be with, and we got along all right.

Pete: That's good. Sis?

Elizabeth: Yes, Bro?

Pete: I have been thinking about all those times—what I did, what I said when I was stubborn, when I was better.

Elizabeth: Bro, you also had periods of depression, especially after Mom died. You went into yourself, and it seemed no one could reach you. That made me sad too.

Pete: Sis, that's true. I was very sad and didn't know how to get unsad.

Elizabeth: What did you try?

Pete: Mostly I just stayed by myself and waited.

Elizabeth: They did give you medicine to help.

Pete: Yes, maybe it helped, but I took a lot of medicines, so I don't know. And there were some people who helped me feel better, but, Sis, I have to tell you a big thing.

Elizabeth: Okay, Bro.

Pete: Much of my life I was pretty much by myself. I couldn't really talk about what bothered me. I couldn't really say well what it was, and I didn't really have someone to tell. Oh, there was Mom. She helped a little. And that woman in Philadelphia. She helped some, but I didn't really have close friends. Even you, Sis—you watched out for me, but I couldn't really tell you either of the things that troubled me.

Elizabeth: You told me of the puppets. And they were a comfort, weren't they?

Pete: Well, yes, sort of, but they were puppets, not people. Mainly, most of the time, it was just too hard to explain.

Elizabeth: Yes, Bro. I guess I can see that. But you know, Bro, that is true for many people. We do all live lives that are sometimes very lonely, even though it might look otherwise. Was there something good, like any learning that came out of that isolation?

Pete: Hard to say, Sis. I did get sort of accustomed to it, even if it wasn't nice. We can talk more about this some other time.

DECEMBER 6, 2020

Elizabeth: I am ready to write in the protection and wisdom of Divine Light and Love.

Pete: Hi, Sis. I am here and happy and busy, but not too busy. Sis?

Elizabeth: Yes, Bro?

Pete: I like you. I love you. You've been a good sister, but Sis, more than just about me, you are a good person. Yes, you have worries. You have flaws, but, my gosh, you have splendors and beauties in your core being.

Elizabeth: Oh, thank you, Bro.

Pete: It's true, Sis. Now I think I can see you more clearly. You are a gem of a person. I was lucky to have you for a sister.

Elizabeth: Aw gee, thanks, Bro.

Pete: You have much you wish to do today. Don't overload yourself. Walk, talk, relax, and take it easy.

Elizabeth: Oh, Pete, I could cry when you say that.

Pete: Go ahead and cry, Sis. It's okay.

Elizabeth: It just so makes me miss you.

Pete: Aw, Sis. Well, I miss you too. But Sis, this place is so amazing, and I am so busy here that I don't have time—time ha ha ha—to wallow in self-pity or grief or regret, even though those are here. Sis?

Elizabeth: Yes, Bro?

Pete: Be kind to yourself most of all. You are a human, learning your own learnings. You've made much of your life. You've done well. Pat yourself on the back. Don't dwell on or exaggerate your failings. Everyone has failings. Yours don't involve hurting anyone else. You have better failings than most. But Sis, you do make attempts to improve. That's good.

Elizabeth: Thanks, Pete. Nice words from you.

Pete: Okay. Just take it easy, Sis. Take good care of your wonderful self.

Elizabeth: You too, Bro.

Pete: Thanks, Sis. Goodbye for now.

D E C E M B E R 3 0 , 2 0 2 0

Elizabeth: I sit to write. Pete, if you are there and wish to talk, I have some questions, and I am ready to write down what you and I say.

Mom: Hello, dear. Pete wants to talk with you.

Elizabeth: Thanks, Mom. Hello, Bro.

Pete: Hi, Sis, it's me. I like talking like this. It's amazing, but you should see where I am. It's even more amazing. Wonderful.

Elizabeth: May I ask you questions about you now and where you are?

Pete: Oh, Question Sister—yes, of course. I'll do my best to answer. Go ahead.

Elizabeth: Okay. Can you say more about who you are now? How are you the same Pete that I know? How are you different?

Pete: Okay, Sis. I'll try, but you might not understand me. I can talk just fine. I guess that's sort of new, but you may not understand the meaning of what I say. I don't look like the brother you know. I don't have the same body. It's different—not heavy, but light. You might not recognize me now by my looks. I know I am me, but it's not about physical appearance. See, that's sort of strange, isn't it?

Elizabeth: Do you have eyes, ears, mouth, hands, legs, and all that?

Pete: Not in the same way.

Elizabeth: But can you see?

Pete: Yes, but not with physical eyes. It's a different kind of knowing. Same with hearing.

Elizabeth: Do you get tired?

Pete: The kind of body I have doesn't get tired as your body might.

Elizabeth: Are there buildings where you are, like houses or schools or businesses?

Pete: Yes, sort of, but that's different too because they are not hard and dense and physical. They are more like ideas of those things. Are you understanding me?

Elizabeth: Sort of, I guess. It does sound different. Are there trees and hills and lakes and streams? Landscapes? Can you see far?

Pete: Oh boy, well, it's the same as people and buildings. Yes and no. Yes, but they are not hard physical landscapes. They are lighter and they can change. It seems almost magical. Things can change easily.

Elizabeth: What makes them change? Can you?

Pete: A little bit, but I'm learning about how it works.

Elizabeth: Oh, I'm trying to see it all.

Pete: Well, Sis, you will when you come, and you'll like it. I know you will. But don't come now. Later, when you have lived all your years and finished what you want to do.

Elizabeth: I'm feeling old and achy now and tired of having to stay at home all the time because of the virus that makes many people get sick and die.

Pete: Well, be careful, Sis. I think you can be careful and be okay. Bye for now, Sis. Bed bug bite. Remember?

Elizabeth: Of course, bed bug bite, Bro.

J A N U A R Y   3 ,   2 0 2 1

Elizabeth: I sit to write. Do you, Pete Bigger Pete have anything to say?

Putty: Hello, dear—your buddy Putty here. How are you?

Elizabeth: I've been having bouts of depression. I'm trying to counteract them. Not serious unless I am in one, which I'm not at the moment.

Putty: Ah, my dear, I am familiar with those, too familiar but not so much now as in my life. Why? Because, to some extent, depression can be related to diet. Stay with fruits, vegetables, and protein. Keep breads, sugars down. They make it worse. Also get your exercise in. You know all this, so let's move on. I'll open the gate.

Elizabeth: Thanks, Putty.

Putty: I can sense you asking me if anyone else calls me Putty. Nope. That is my nickname for you, only you, to call me.

Elizabeth: Oh, okay—thanks.

Putty: Now the door . . .

Pete: Hi, Sis. I'm glad you called. I like talking with you now that I am reviewing my life. I forgot a lot about it. I remember some of the end—when everything was hard.

Elizabeth: Yes, it was.

Pete: But now I am remembering when I was little. I'm trying to remember my birth *and* before.

Why such a life?

Elizabeth: Yes, I'm very curious too.

Pete: Well, I cannot remember that from inside that life, but people here are helping me to remember and reclaim my bigger self—the self that knows all the lives and between—the soul. It seems we come into any one life without remembering anything from before. That doesn't make sense to me, but I am still learning. There is so much to learn.

Elizabeth: Do you know why you were born into the life as Pete, my brother?

Pete: Some was my decision, some suggested to me. I don't really have the whole picture of it yet. I know you are interested.

Elizabeth: Aren't you?

Pete: Yes, but I'm also a bit scared to learn some things I might not want to know because once I learn them, I won't be able to unlearn them. And maybe I won't want to talk about them either, but I'll try to tell you because I know you want to know.

Elizabeth: Thanks, Bro—and Bro, if you learn some difficult things, maybe if you tell me, we can sort out the difficult stuff together. I would do my best.

Pete: Gee thanks, Sis. You are a good sister even now. Take good care of yourself, Sis.

Elizabeth: You too, Bro.

Pete: Good night, Sis. Is it night there now?

Elizabeth: Yes. Is it night where you are?

Pete: It can be, but right now it's sort of in-between. We don't have time like clocks and days and night, but the light, such as it is, can and does change.

Elizabeth: By itself? In some regular ways?

Pete: I'm not sure. But I can always see what's happening even though I don't see with eyes.

Elizabeth: So maybe you don't need light to see like I need light for my eyes to see.

Pete: Something like that, Sis. Bye, Sis.

Elizabeth: Bye, Bro.

JANUARY 6, 2021

Elizabeth: I sit to write. Pete Bigger Pete, are you talkable? I'm feeling better.

Putty: Hello, dear one. I hope this is the beginning of a better year for you. It's time for that, yes?

Elizabeth: Yes, and for many people. Is there a lesson for humans from the viruses? I wonder.

Putty: Well, well, you certainly have a curious and open mind. Let's open the door.

Pete: Hi, Sis—it's Pete <u>and</u> Bigger Pete. We're more together now.

Elizabeth: I'm sure I don't understand, but hello to you both or the one you now are together.

Pete: Sis (I'll call you that still), I am fine. I am still learning about this place and about me and the life I just had. Sis?

Elizabeth: Yes, Bro?

Pete: I like living in this place that is so full of love. It's like instead of air, there is love. It's amazing. And Sis?

Elizabeth: Yes, Bro?

Pete: Because there isn't time—no nights, no days—there is a different feel about everything.

This part is hard to tell, but it is an easy feeling. I'm losing my sense of time I might have had on Earth, even though I didn't bother much with time there, especially at the end. But even as little a time sense as I had, it was something of a habit that is irrelevant now. The effect is lovely—calm, reassuring, easy. And Sis, imagine breathing love instead of air. Oh, Sis, when you come, you'll see. But I know you're not coming yet, so we can talk this way until then. For now, take good care of your wonderful self. And call on me again.

Elizabeth: Yes, Bro. Bye for now.

JANUARY 14, 2021

Elizabeth: Here I am, ready to write.

Putty: Hello, dear one. Good for you to do this.

Elizabeth: How can I be in touch with spirit in other ways?

Putty: Ah, yes, you can. You need to call, then be quiet and listen. Wait and then write what you think you hear rather than having it all bypass that to go through your arm. But you are very good with your arm, so don't give this up. Now, ready for the voices at the gate?

Elizabeth: Yes, thank you, Putty.

Mom: Hello, dear. Pete? Yes, he's here for a moment. Pete, you speak first. It's Elizabeth calling.

Pete: Hi, Sis.

Elizabeth: Hi, Bro. How are you? What are you busy with? Anything you can tell me?

Pete: Sis, I am sorry you and the others were older. You all grew up and went away.

As Pete was the youngest of five children, we four older siblings grew up before he did and left home while he was still small.

Elizabeth: Yes, Bro. What did that mean for you?

Pete: It made me lonely. And when I went away, I was lonely too. Actually, I was very lonely most of my life. I liked it when people stayed close. But so many left, and it seemed they left *me*. I didn't leave them. Sis?

Elizabeth: Yes, Bro?

Pete: What was I like as a boy?

Elizabeth: You were a lot of fun. You liked to play. You liked reading books. You were a joy to be with. You could be stubborn but mostly a good kid.

Pete: Oh, good.

Elizabeth: What do you think?

Pete: Sis, I didn't have close friends. And when someone wanted to get close with me, I didn't want to because maybe they'd leave.

Elizabeth: Well, Bro, that's true. No guarantees. Things change in life. People move, go away, change jobs. Some die. Life can be lonely. And Bro, friends usually share lots of talking, and talking was not always easy for you.

Pete: True, Sis. I liked to be by myself a lot. It was easier, didn't have to talk or think too hard. Lots of time in my room by myself. And when I was sad, being by myself was much easier.

Elizabeth: Wow, Bro, you have been thinking of your life.

Pete: Yes, Sis. A lot.

Elizabeth: Okay, Bro.

JANUARY 17, 2021

Elizabeth: Here I am, ready to write in the protection and wisdom of Divine Light and Love. Pete Bigger Pete?

Putty: Hello, dear one—this is your Putty, ready to open the door. First, I give you a big bear hug and hope you can feel such a hug.

Elizabeth: I get chills.

Putty: Ah.

Elizabeth: Just the thought of it. I wish I could have met you. I think I would have liked that very much.

Putty: Me as well, but we do have this.

Elizabeth: True. And it is special indeed.

Putty: Yes. The door?

Elizabeth: Yes, please, Putty. Who is there?

Pete: Hi, Sis—it's Pete and Bigger Pete together.

Elizabeth: How are you, Bro?

Pete: Fine, Sis. Are you doing the book?

Elizabeth: Slowly, yes.

Pete: Okay, Sis, but do it soon. I want people to read the book, so it's good to finish it soon.

Elizabeth: Okay, Bro.

JANUARY 19, 2021

Elizabeth: I open my heart and thank you all. Why all these dreams? Geez! Anyway, I am ready to write. I light my candle and wait. I feel forces at work that I do not understand. Can anyone tell me anything?

Putty: Hello, dear one. So glad when you come to speak with us. Yes, forces are at work. There always are, but some may be felt more than others or by you more than others or at some time more than others. You need not worry. Just do your usual things. Do keep this line open though because this is <u>your</u> connection, and those in spirit who wish to speak can then do so.

Elizabeth: Thank you, Putty.

Putty: You know what to do. Do walk as you have been doing. Get enough rest. This allows communication too, even if you do not remember it. You're on the right path. The forces you sense are strong and will have an impact, but not directly on you. Keep your quiet life. It is good and helps provide balance to craziness elsewhere. And, if you're wondering, I have had help on this answer. Others are speaking through me.

Elizabeth: Yes, I was wondering. Thanks.

Putty: Now others may wish to speak.

Pete: Hi, Sis.

Elizabeth: Pete, Bro, how are you? I'm glad to hear from you. Is this talking this way together okay with you for now?

Pete: Yes, of course, Sis.

Elizabeth: I don't want to be pulling you away from what you want or need to do where you are now.

Pete: It's fine, especially while you are working on the book. Do work on it.

Elizabeth: I am, Bro. Please make any suggestions or additions you wish to.

Pete: I'll tell you one right now, Sis—a big one. Be sure you have in the book for people <u>not</u> to be afraid of death. A long, painful death is not nice, of course, and death out of war or hatred is not good, but *after* death, it is all fine.

Elizabeth: For everyone all the time?

Pete: Well, Sis, that is a wise question. But for most, to come to the end of a good life and pass quietly away out of that life is not a bad thing. Because this afterlife anyway is lovely. I mean by "lovely" it is full of love. Love everywhere. It is the work of those on Earth to learn how to live in such love, to love others even when those others seem undeserving. Love is not a prize. Love is.

Elizabeth: That is very wise, Bro.

Pete: I think, Sis, I have become wiser little by little.

Elizabeth: You were always wise, Bro. It's just that a few things got in the way of others seeing it.

Pete: Ah, Sis.

Elizabeth: True, Bro. It took me a very long time, and it surprises me now and delights me how very wise you are.

Pete: Oh, Sis. Call again soon.

J A N U A R Y   2 0 ,   2 0 2 1

Elizabeth: I open my heart, light my candle, and thank you all. I would be delighted to hear from any who wish to speak. What does all that love feel like? Any advice for us Earthlings now?

Let me drop into a space or rise into a space where my hand can write your words.

Putty: Hello, my dear one. I am here and ready to open the door.

Elizabeth: Oh, thank you as always, Putty.

Putty: Write fast. Many are here.

Mom: Hello, dear. I'm glad you've been careful through this pandemic and all the tribulations. Continue that. There are others here. I'll say goodbye.

Elizabeth: Thanks, Mom.

Unidentified voices: Hello, dear daughter of Earth. You so want to know everything. The biggest advice is for those on Earth to realize we are all one and to love others as yourself. But if the behavior is too egregious, then avoid any contact that would be hateful. Do not wish ill on others, much as you might wish. See instead how you can find something to appreciate. And if you can only see horrors you would hate, acknowledge how you might have traces of those qualities or thoughts or behavior like that in yourself. In other words, be as kind as you can be. And keep up the effort to be patient with the foibles of others <u>and</u> of yourself.

Elizabeth: Whew! That is excellent advice. Not new, but always a good reminder.

J A N U A R Y   2 1 ,   2 0 2 1

Elizabeth: Here I am. I was interrupted yesterday. I open my heart now, light my candle, and thank you all in the protection and wisdom of Divine Light and Love.

Putty: Hello, dear Elizabeth—this is Putty, your Putty. I am putty in your hands.

Elizabeth: Haha—funny!

Putty: I'll open the door, okay?

Elizabeth: Yes, please, Putty, and thank you.

Pete: Hi, Sis.

Elizabeth: Oh, Bro, how are you?

Pete: I'm fine, Sis—as fine as can be. How are you?

Elizabeth: I'm okay and glad to talk with you.

Pete: Do you have questions, Question Sister?

Elizabeth: Yes. A big one. Are you ready?

Pete: Yes, Sis. Go ahead.

Elizabeth: What kind of choice did you have to come into the life on Earth as Peter? Did you choose to be male? To have our family? To have Down syndrome? To be who you became?

Pete: Oh, Sis, I know you want to know, to have answers, but I cannot tell you the whole story yet. I am still learning it myself. Here is what I can tell you now.

I did have some choice to have the challenges I did. What I mean is it isn't about the family, the birthdate exactly, the sex, the Down syndrome. By the way, I have no Down syndrome now. The choices had more to do with what life lessons I might learn. I told you about the dependence one, that that was something of a choice, and that's a big one. But how any particulars of a life would provide that experience, I did <u>not</u> set out in any list of requirements. That may not be the answer you were looking for, but it is more about how things actually work, or, I should say, at least worked for me. I suspect there are grand variations on the plan.

Maybe this will help. Suppose you are hungry and go to a restaurant or a grocery store to find food. The hunger motivates you, but what you decide to eat depends on what is available at the time and place when you go to look. So, in choosing a life, it wasn't about choosing all the details but about a purpose or purposes for life experience. Does this make sense?

Elizabeth: Yes, Bro, you are explaining clearly, and I thank you. And Bro, I may end up asking the same question but only because my memory isn't great. I sometimes forget things.

Pete: Oh, Sis, I don't know why I say this but, somehow, I want to say to you to drink more water.

Elizabeth: Okay, Bro. Thanks.

Pete: You are welcome. Have a good day, Sis, and good writing. Bed bug bite.

Elizabeth: Bed bug bite.

J A N U A R Y   2 7 ,   2 0 2 1

Elizabeth: I am eager to hear from anyone about anything. I am ready. My arm writes on its own. Whose words?

Unidentified voices: We are here in support of you and your work. Fine work it is.

Elizabeth: Anything to add?

Unidentified voices: Well, dear one, let's see if your dear brother has something to say.

Pete: Hi, Sis. I'm glad you called for me. I wish I could tell you all about here.

Elizabeth: You keep saying it's amazing. Do you miss your old body?

Pete: Not at all. It did as much as it could, but, well, that wasn't great, especially at the end.

Elizabeth: Did you want to live longer?

Pete: No! I was just not sure how to leave that life, how to do it, what it would feel like. Imagine leaving everyone and everything you know to go somewhere unknown.

Elizabeth: But you had visited your afterlife, the other side of life. Isn't it now as you saw it before?

Pete: Yes and no. It was always lovely, but I didn't have the full picture before. Now that I am here, I am fully here, and I get to see and experience the full thing. You'll see.

Elizabeth: Is there anything you think I might not like?

Pete: Hmm, I don't know—hard to say. I think you'll like it, but you wouldn't like it now because there is work that you want to finish. You've been here with me (when you are sleeping), but then you go back.

Elizabeth: I wish I could remember.

Pete: Part of you does. Enough of you does so you can tell when anyone's description hits a false note. People experience here differently, but when you come, I think you'll like it.

Elizabeth: Bro, how should I end the book?

Pete: With a thank you to everyone and a giggle.

JANUARY 28, 2021

Elizabeth: I am open. I would be delighted to hear any messages or guidance.

Pete: Hi, Sis. Oh, I wish you could be here and seeing this place with me. It is beautiful. There is always lovely music, a special kind. And it smells nice here too. Not flowers or perfume. It must be the scent of love.

Elizabeth: Ooooh, Bro, that's beautiful.

Pete: I don't know what to tell you. You're the writer, but I'm the one that's here. I miss you.

Sis?

Elizabeth: Yes, Bro?

Pete: You're a good sister. Maybe we'll have other lives together.

Elizabeth: I don't know, Bro. Let me finish this one. It may be enough. Life isn't easy.

Pete: Yours wasn't bad, Sis. Mine wasn't too bad. Sis?

Elizabeth: Yes, Bro?

Pete: I don't have anything else to say now. I just like talking with you.

Elizabeth: Me too, Bro. I'm going to sleep shortly.

Pete: Okay, Sis. Sleep tight. Bed bug bite.

J A N U A R Y   3 1 ,   2 0 2 1

Elizabeth: I am ready to write.

Pete: Hi, Sis. I am here in my new special place.

Elizabeth: Tell me about it.

Pete: Oh, Sis, it's a soft place. There are edges of things, but not hard, solid, difficult edges. Everything is easy, so easy. I don't understand how it can be so nice, all the time nice. Why can't life on Earth, where you are, where I was, be like this?

Elizabeth: Good question, Bro. I don't know the answer. Maybe that is what we are supposed to do with our lives—make where we live better.

Pete: But Sis, this place where I am is already nice—beautiful, really.

Elizabeth: I was talking about where I am, where people can be mean, where there is war, disease, poverty, hatred, and all that.

Pete: Oh yeah, Sis—I'm not there anymore.

Elizabeth: And Bro, your life wasn't always so lovely, especially at the end.

Pete: Thanks for helping me get through that.

Elizabeth: Of course, Bro, my dear sweet Bro. I'm glad you're in a good place now. What does it look like?

Pete: Well, Sis, hard to say. There's a lot that sort of looks the same, but, oh, how can I tell it? It's just softer, not so hard, not so hurtful, not dirty, not a lot of problems. I told you about the music. It's not really a humming. It's not really voices singing or pianos or trumpets, but I'd have to call it music. It's sound, and it changes, and it's lovely to listen to if you want to listen to it.

Elizabeth: Do you eat?

Pete: No, not really. I mean, you can if you want but probably more out of habit or curiosity because we don't have bodies that need food. No need to eat.

Elizabeth: That's different.

Pete: Well, you <u>can</u> eat if you want, but there's no need. No getting hungry.

Elizabeth: What does it smell like?

Pete: Oh, let me see. Now, I haven't really noticed. I mean, there's nothing really smelly. It doesn't smell bad. There's not much smell, but now that you mention it, I'm paying attention.

There is a nice smell around where I am now.

Elizabeth: Maybe you are what smells nice, Bro!

Pete: Aw, Sis. It's kind of a faint sweet smell, pleasant but not strong. I don't think I am really smelling like I would smell with a nose before. It's sort of thought or the remembrance of smell maybe. Sis, it's hard to say. I don't think I'm describing it well.

Elizabeth: Well, does it always smell the same, or have you noticed different smells at different times or in different places?

Pete: Sis, I guess I haven't really been noticing, so I can't describe it well.

Elizabeth: That's okay, Bro. I'm just trying to understand what it's like where you are.

Pete: Yeah, Sis, I know. Question Sister. Here's the important part. It's beautiful and the whole place is love, and I am free and happy to be here. I wish you could be here yourself. Your questions would be answered. We could be together and enjoy it all together. I know you are not coming now. But you'll see when you come, whenever you do, a long time from now.

Elizabeth: That's right, Bro. I am curious, have lots of questions, but I hope to live many more years to finish my life here first. When I do come, I hope I can see you and you can show me everything.

Pete: Sounds good, Sis. Sis?

Elizabeth: Yes, Bro?

Pete: What are you doing?

Elizabeth: Right now, I am sitting writing our words with my yellow pencil on my yellow pad of striped paper. I am sitting on my bed in my house, and I am sort of half-asleep in a trance. But what I am working on in the days is the Bigger Pete book.

Pete: Oh, Sis, I am so glad. That's cool, Sis. Finish it well. Send it out, and when you do, send it out with love. Put love in all the pages so people can have all the love.

Elizabeth: Oh, Bro, that's beautiful.

Pete: Well then, Sis, shall we say goodbye for now?

Elizabeth: Yes, Bro—goodbye for now.

Pete: Call me again, Sis. I love you. Bed bug bite.

Elizabeth: Bed bug bite, Bro. I love you too. Anything else?

Pete: Yes, remember the part about the love. That's most important. Love, love, love, love, love.

ABOUT THE AUTHOR

Elizabeth Bodien is the author of two books of poetry: *Blood, Metal, Fiber, Rock* and *Oblique Music: A Book of Hours* and one nonfiction work: *Journeys with Fortune: A Tale of Other Lives*, a collection of her past lives experienced while in hypnotic trance. Her poems, essays, and book reviews have appeared in *Cimarron Review*, *Crannóg*, and *Parabola*, among other publications in the USA, Ireland, Canada, Australia, and India. She holds degrees in cultural anthropology, consciousness studies, religions, and poetry, and has worked as an English instructor in Japan, an organic farmer in the Oregon mountains, a childbirth instructor in West Africa, a Montessori teacher, and as a professor of cultural anthropology. Bodien, who grew up in the "burned over" district of western New York, now lives near Hawk Mountain, Pennsylvania, USA.

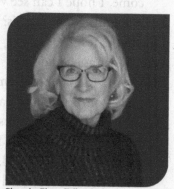

Photo by Elaine Zelker, LLC